P. Johnson

P. Johnson

Clinical Pharmacology of the Beta-Adrenoceptor Blocking Drugs

Clinical Pharmacology of the Beta-Adrenoceptor Blocking Drugs

William H. Frishman, M.D.

Associate Professor of Medicine
Director of the Heart Station
Albert Einstein College of Medicine
Bronx, New York

Teaching Scholar of The American Heart Association

foreword by

Edmund H. Sonnenblick, M.D.

Professor of Medicine
Chief, Division of Cardiology
Albert Einstein College of Medicine
Bronx, New York

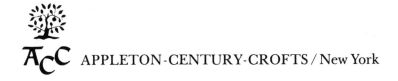
APPLETON-CENTURY-CROFTS / New York

81 82 83 84 / 10 9 8 7 6 5 4 3 2

Library of Congress Catalog Card Number: 80-23702

Prentice-Hall International, Inc., London
Prentice-Hall of Australia, Pty. Ltd., Sydney
Prentice-Hall of India Private Limited, New Delhi
Prentice-Hall of Japan, Inc., Tokyo
Prentice-Hall of Southeast Asia (Pte.) Ltd., Singapore
Whitehall Books Ltd., Wellington, New Zealand

Library of Congress Cataloging in Publication Data

Frishman, William H.   1946–
    Clinical pharmacology of the Beta-adrenoceptor blocking drugs.

Includes index.
    1. Adrenergic beta receptor blockaders.   I. Title.
[DNLM: 1. Adrenergic beta blockaders.   2. Cardiovascular diseases — Drug
therapy.   QV132 F917c]
RM323.5.F74   615'.71   80-23702
ISBN 0-8385-1143-0

PRINTED IN THE UNITED STATES OF AMERICA

To my wife, Esther Rose;
my children, Sheryl and Amy;
and to the memory of
Aaron H. Frishman,
father, teacher, and friend

CONTRIBUTORS

Ronald M. Becker, M.D.
   Assistant Professor of Surgery, Division of Cardiothoracic Surgery, Albert Einstein
   College of Medicine, Bronx, New York

Richard Davis, M.D.
   Division of Cardiology, Albert Einstein College of Medicine, Bronx, New York

Edward Eisenberg, M.D.
   Department of Medicine, Albert Einstein College of Medicine, Bronx, New York

Uri Elkayam, M.D.
   Assistant Professor of Medicine, Division of Cardiology, University of California
   at Irvine, School of Medicine and Medical Center, Orange, California

Robert W.B. Frater, M.B., Ch.B., M.S.
   Professor of Surgery and Chief, Division of Cardiothoracic Surgery,
   Albert Einstein College of Medicine, Bronx, New York

Stanley Halprin, M.D.
   Division of Cardiology, Albert Einstein College of Medicine, Bronx, New York

Maryhelen Hossler, R.N.
   Division of Cardiology, Rutgers University College of Medicine,
   Raritan Valley Hospital, Piscataway, New Jersey

Harold Jacob, M.D.
   Department of Medicine, Albert Einstein College of Medicine, Bronx, New York

Alan Kadish, M.D.
   Department of Medicine, Peter Bent Brigham Hospital, Boston, Massachusetts

Marc Kirschner, M.D.

Division of Cardiology, Albert Einstein College of Medicine, Bronx, New York

John Kostis, M.D.

Associate Professor of Medicine and Director of the Cardiac Catheterization Lab, Rutgers University College of Medicine, Raritan Valley Hospital, Piscataway, New Jersey

Masayuki Matsumoto, M.D., Ph.D.

Visiting Professor of Medicine, Division of Cardiology, Albert Einstein College of Medicine, Bronx, New York; Associate Professor of Medicine, University of Osaka, Osaka, Japan

Yasu Oka, M.D.

Associate Professor of Anesthesiology, Department of Anesthesiology, Albert Einstein College of Medicine, Bronx, New York

Louis Orkin, M.D.

Professor and Chairman, Department of Anesthesiology, Albert Einstein College of Medicine, Bronx, New York

Hillel Ribner, M.D.

Assistant Professor of Medicine, Northwestern University School of Medicine, Chicago, Illinois

Ralph Silverman, M.D.

Assistant Professor of Medicine, Albert Einstein College of Medicine, Bronx, New York

Edmund H. Sonnenblick, M.D.

Professor of Medicine and Chief, Division of Cardiology, Albert Einstein College of Medicine, Bronx, New York

Morris Stampfer, M.D.

Clinical Associate Professor of Medicine, Division of Cardiology, Albert Einstein College of Medicine, Bronx, New York

Joel Strom, M.D.

Assistant Professor of Medicine, Co-Director Non-Invasive Cardiac Labs, Division of Cardiology, Albert Einstein College of Medicine, Bronx, New York

Jerome Weinstein, M.D.

Consultant in Clinical Pharmacology, St. Vincent's Hospital and Medical Center, New York, New York

CONTENTS

PREFACE

THE INTRODUCTION OF β-adrenoceptor blocking drugs to clinical medicine has provided the most significant advance in the medical management of cardiovascular diseases during the past 20 years. While the original investigators envisioned these agents for the treatment of patients with angina pectoris, hypertension, and arrhythmias, their therapeutic benefits have extended well beyond the cardiovascular sphere. For instance, the β-blockers have been utilized in the treatment of porphyria, acne vulgaris, and a host of neuropsychiatric conditions. No group of synthetic drugs have had such widespread applicability in human pharmacotherapy.

Although the competitive inhibition of a β-adrenoceptor is a simple pharmacologic concept, there are many unsettled issues regarding the molecular and clinical pharmacology of these drugs. There are a host of β-adrenergic blocking agents that are now being marketed worldwide. These agents have similarities and differences that have clinical relevance. Thousands of scientific articles have been written about these drugs. This bulk of knowledge has never been synthesized for the clinician's easy reference. This book was conceived to organize this plethora of knowledge.

The controversies and questions involving the β-blocking drugs and their pharmacodynamic and pharmacokinetic differences are discussed. The clinical applications of these agents and their adverse reactions are reviewed in detail. Special chapters deal with the problems of overdose, and the use of these drugs in surgery and pre- and postmyocardial infarction. Specific drugs are discussed in detail based on the author's personal experiences in order to illustrate how chemical and pharmacokinetic differences can influence the therapeutic applications of these agents. The final chapter concludes with the changing concepts in adrenergic molecular pharmacology and extrapolates this new knowledge to disease and pharmacotherapy.

This book is directed to the teachers and students of adrenergic pharmacology (undergraduate and postgraduate), whether they be in general medicine, basic science, research cardiology, anesthesiology, surgery, pediatrics, psychology, pharmacy, toxicology, and epidemiology, and particularly to all clinicians who use β-blockers in daily medical practice.

The list of people and organizations to whom I am indebted directly or indirectly for helping me complete my work would easily fill an entire page. I want to start with my mother and father. The memory of my father who died from premature coronary artery disease inspired my interest in cardiovascular medicine and pharmacology.

It is hardly possible to acknowledge the many medical students, house officers, and cardiac fellows from whom I absorbed many ideas and who have served indispensable roles as collaborators, critics, supporters, and constant sources of stimulation.

To my devoted and loyal secretary, Nina Scotti, a special tribute: it was on her very capable shoulders that an immense amount of work fell. Her patience, good humor, skill, and unremitting labors deserve more thanks than I can ever provide.

On the medical side, I should like to begin with Dr. Thomas Killip, III, who gave me the opportunity to work in adult cardiology and encouraged my early research endeavors in cardiovascular pharmacology. I wish to express my sincere thanks to Dr. Edmund Sonnenblick for his critical review of the manuscript and the constant support and encouragement he has given me.

I wish to thank my professional colleagues at the Albert Einstein College of Medicine and the New York Hospital-Cornell Medical Center who were my collaborators in research and in preparation of this book.

I will always be grateful to the American Heart Association who chose me as their "Teaching Scholar" enabling me to pursue my interests in medical education. Education of my colleagues and students was the primary motivation for writing this book. I also wish to thank the National Heart-Lung Institute (HL-00653-1) who have supported my efforts in preventive cardiology, of which β-adrenoceptor blockade has and will play an important role.

I wish to acknowledge my appreciation for the efforts of Albert Nitzburg and Marcia Poland for their editorial reviews. I am particularly grateful to my editor, Robert E. McGrath of Appleton-Century-Crofts, for his expert guidance in the preparation of this volume.

In many ways, my most important collaborators were my wife, Esther, and my two daughters, Sheryl and Amy, whose patience, devotion, and forebearance were commendable and whose confidence in the outcome of my efforts was far greater than mine.

Bronx, New York
March 1980

FOREWORD

DETAILED PHARMACOLOGIC KNOWLEDGE stands alone as a basic science, but successful pharmacotherapy requires application of this information to disease-induced abnormalities in individual patients. The concept that catecholamines mediate their effects by stimulating specific cellular receptors provided one of the most significant advances in basic pharmacology. The subsequent discovery of compounds that could competitively block these receptors and thus interfere with catecholamines was not only an important pharmacologic advance, but probably contributed to the most exciting breakthrough in human therapeutics during the past 20 years: the discovery of β-adrenoceptor blocking drugs.

The early investigators in the field of catecholamine pharmacology, Ahlquist, Black, Powell, Slater, Lands, and others, conceived β-adrenoceptor blocking drugs for the treatment of angina pectoris. The applications of these drugs in cardiovascular practice today have extended to the management of patients with arrhythmias, hypertension, congenital heart disease, myocardial infarction, mitral valve prolapse, hypertrophic cardiomyopathy, and aortic dissection. Additionally, these agents are now widely prescribed by neurologists for migraines, by ophthalmologists for glaucoma, by psychiatrists, dermatologists, gastroenterologists, endocrinologists, anesthesiologists, and gynecologists. The list of noncardiac indications continues to grow. There are no group of synthetic compounds in the history of human pharmacotherapy that have had such widespread applicability. Only the naturally occurring corticosteroids have had more use in treatment of disease.

The competitive inhibition of a β-adrenoceptor is a simple pharmacologic concept, and since the discovery of propranolol there has been an explosion of the β-blocking drugs on the world scene. Now there are drugs that inhibit β-adrenoceptors in the heart and periphery (nonselective). There are drugs that completely block β-receptors in the heart, and spare peripheral and bronchial β-adrenoceptors (cardioselective). There are drugs that have partial agonist effects (intrinsic sympathomimetic activity), drugs with quinidinelike actions (membrane-stabilizing property), and a β-adrenoceptor blocking drug that also has α-adrenergic blocking activity. There are drugs with varying degrees of protein-binding and lipid solubility. Certain compounds are metabolized in the liver, some have active metabolites, some excreted unchanged in the urine. Pharmacologic half-life and bioavailability vary from compound to compound. These pharmacodynamic and pharmacokinetic differences may have important ramifications in therapy patient compliance, and adverse drug reactions.

With this growing body of knowledge, a compendium has become necessary that could organize the vast literature and clinical experience of the β-adrenoceptor blockers.

Dr. Frishman has risen to this challenge and succeeded by writing a most comprehensive and thorough text on the β-adrenoceptor blocking drugs. He is especially well qualified for this task. He is an accomplished physician-scientist who has personally worked with most of the β-adrenoceptor blockers in clinical trials. His original contributions include the first demonstration of the platelet-inhibiting actions of propranolol and the utility of noninvasive cardiac evaluation in assessing comparative drug activity. His large personal experience with propranolol, metoprolol, pindolol, and labetolol provides an immediacy as well as authority to this presentation.

Dr. Frishman, an enthusiastic and skillful teacher, and his contributors have organized and communicated difficult pharmacologic and physiologic concepts. Moreover, the application of this material in clinical situations has been clearly presented. Students of adrenergic pharmacology will easily comprehend this text. However, the compelling achievement of this text is that after reading the following pages, the physician-therapist will gain a comprehensive understanding of the β-adrenoceptor blocking drugs and the scientific basis for their use in clinical practice.

Edmund H. Sonnenblick, M.D.
Professor of Medicine
Chief, Division of Cardiology
Albert Einstein College of Medicine
Bronx, New York

CHAPTER ONE

Pharmacodynamic and Pharmacokinetic Properties

William H. Frishman

T HE findings that the relative potency of a series of sympathomimetic amines varied with the effector organs or systems led Ahlquist,[1] in 1948, to conclude that there were two distinct types of adrenergic receptors, which he classified as α- and β-receptors. The distribution of these receptors is given in Table 1-1, which shows some of the responses produced by activation of these receptors. β-Adrenoreceptors have been subsequently further divided into two main groups: β_1-receptors in the heart; and β_2-receptors in the bronchi and blood vessels.[2-4]

TABLE 1-1. **Distribution of Adrenoceptors**

Organ	Receptor	Effect of Stimulation
Heart	β_1	Increase in heart rate
	β_1	Increase in cardiac contractility
	β_1	Accelerate AV conduction
Bronchi	β_2	Dilatation
Blood vessels	β_2	Dilatation
	α	Constriction
Eye	α	Dilatation of pupil
Gastrointestinal tract	α, β	Reduction in motility

Until the discovery of dichloroisoprenaline (DCI), by Powell and Slater[5] in 1958, Ahlquist's theories were the subject of a great deal of skepticism. The discovery that DCI selectively blocked responses which, according to Ahlquist, were mediated by β-receptors, has proven to be one of the most exciting developments in human pharmacology.

The β-blocking agents developed after DCI, by the pioneering work of Black,[6] were initially conceived of as a means of treating angina pectoris. It soon became clear, however, that β-blocking agents had much to offer in other clinical settings. The application of these agents has been accelerated by the development of drugs possessing a degree of selectivity for various subgroups of the β-receptor population. More controversial has been the introduction of agents with varying degrees of intrinsic sympathomimetic activity (agonist effect).

Although a useful range of β-blocking drugs is now available to the clinician in most western countries, only propranolol, nadolol, metoprolol, and timolol are approved by the Food and Drug Administration (FDA) for clinical use in the United States. Other β-blockers have yet to be marketed in the United States because final FDA approval requires submission of both long-term animal and human studies. These extraordinary requirements are based on questions of safety raised by the tumorigenicity of some of these agents (practolol and alprenolol), and the severe cutaneous ocular peritoneal syndrome seen with practolol.[7-9] The carcinogenicity study requirements have been met for many of these newer β-blockers (acebutolol, atenolol, metoprolol, nadolol, pindolol, oxprenolol labetalol, and timolol) and long-term studies of these agents are now in progress in the United States.[7]

Most of the β-blockers presently under study in the United States, and/ or marketed abroad, appear to have virtually the same range of effects as does propranolol. However, differences in metabolism, passage through the blood-brain barrier, direct effects on membranes, and degreees of intrinsic sympathomimetic activity may ultimately prove clinically meaningful.

In this chapter, the pharmacodynamic and pharmacokinetic properties of the newer β-blockers will be discussed, and comparisons with propranolol and practolol will be provided.

DIFFERENCES IN PHARMACODYNAMIC PROPERTIES (TABLE 1-2)

All of the β-blocking drugs are specific antagonists.[10] Thus, stimulation of β-adrenoreceptors in the heart, irrespective of the manner in which that stimulation is evoked, can be blocked by β-adrenergic blockers. However, the response to agents that stimulate contractility of the heart by other pathways, such as calcium or digitalis, is unaffected.

β-BLOCKING POTENCY

β-Blocking drugs are competitive inhibitors of the effects of catecholamines at β-adrenoreceptor sites. They reduce the effect of any concentration of agonist on a sensitive tissue. This occurs in such a way that the dose-response curve is shifted to the right: a given tissue response then requires a higher concentration of agonist in the presence of the drug. β-blocking potency is judged by the inhibition of the tachycardia produced by isoproterenol.[11] As shown in Table 1-2, mg for mg, pindolol and timolol are the most potent, and acebutolol, alprenolol, practolol, and sotalol are the least potent of the β-blocking agents.[11]

TABLE 1–2.   Some Differences in Pharmacologic Properties among β-Adrenoreceptor Blocking Drugs

Drug	Synonyms	β-blockade potency ratio (propranolol = 1)	Cardio-selectivity	Partial agonist activity	Membrane-stabilizing activity
Acebutolol	Sectral	0.3	+	+	+
Alprenolol	M & B 17, 803A H56/26	0.3	0	+ +	+
	Aptin				
	Betaptin				
	Betacard				
Atenolol	ICI66082	1.0	+	0	0
	Tenormin				
Metoprolol	H93/26	1.0	+	0	±
	Lopresor				
	Betaloc				
Oxprenolol	Ciba 39089 Ba	0.5-1.0	0	+ +	+
	Trasicor				
Pindolol	LB46	6.0	0	+ + +	+
	Visken				
Practolol	ICI50172	0.3	+	+ +	0
	Eraldin				
Propranolol	ICI45520	1.0	0	0	+ +
	Inderal Avlocardin				
Sotalol	MJ1999	0.3	0	0	0
	Betacardone				
	Sotacor				
Timolol	MK-950	6.0	0	±	0
	Blocadren				
Isomer: D-Propranolol		0.1	0	0	+ +

From Waal-Manning HJ[11]

STRUCTURE-ACTIVITY RELATIONSHIP

The chemical structures of β-adrenergic blocking agents (Fig. 1-1) have several features in common with isoproterenol. The 2-C side chain, with an alkyl substituted secondary or tertiary amine, seems to determine the affinity for the β-receptor.[12] The larger the alkyl group, the greater the affinity for the β-receptor.[13] The particular structure attaches to the receptor site, and the nature of the substituents on the aromatic ring determines whether the effects will be predominantly activation or blockade.[12] The configuration of the asymmetric β carbon of the side chain is crucial for pharmacologic activity. β-Blocking drugs exist as pairs of optical isomers. Almost all of the blocking activity resides in the levorotatory isomer, however. For propranolol[14] and alprenolol[15] the (−) levorotatory isomers are up to 100 times more active than the (+) dextrorotatory isomers. Only the racemic mixture of each drug, consisting of equal parts of the two isomers, is available for clinical use. The different stereoisomers of β-adrenergic blocking drugs are useful for differentiation between the effects of β-receptor and nonspecific properties (i.e., local anesthetic properties possessed by both forms) but, clinically, the (+) dextrorotatory isomers are of no clinical value (see Table 1-2).

MEMBRANE-STABILIZING ACTIVITY

Membrane-stabilizing activity, sometimes referred to as a "quinidine-like" effect, or "local anesthetic" action, is unrelated to competitive inhibition of catecholamine action and is exhibited equally by the two optical isomers of the drug.[12] These properties were originally defined electrophysiologically: propranolol,[14] oxprenolol,[16] alprenolol,[15] and acebutolol[17] all reduce the rate of rise of the intracardiac action potential, without affecting the overall duration of the spike or the resting potential. The concentration of propranolol at which this effect has been demonstrated, in vitro, with human ventricular muscle, is approximately 50 to 100 times the propranolol blood level associated with the inhibition of exercise-induced tachycardia.[18] With other β-blockers, the difference is even greater, and it is unlikely that plasma levels associated with "quinidinelike" effects are clinically significant.[19] The antiarrhythmic effects of these drugs have been shown to be due to β-blockade, unrelated to the membrane-stabilizing effect.[20] Practolol, which is without membrane effects, is as effective an antiarrhythmic agent as propranolol (with membrane properties) in equipotent doses.[20]

INTRINSIC SYMPATHOMIMETIC ACTIVITY (ISA)

β-Blockers, by definition, antagonize the action of agonists on the β-adrenoreceptor. Of the β-blocking drugs listed in Table 1-2, propranolol, sotalol, timolol, atenolol, and metoprolol cause no observable effect when they interact with β-receptors in the absence of a primary agonist, such as epinephrine or isoproterenol.[12] Paradoxically, the others (acebutolol, alprenolol,

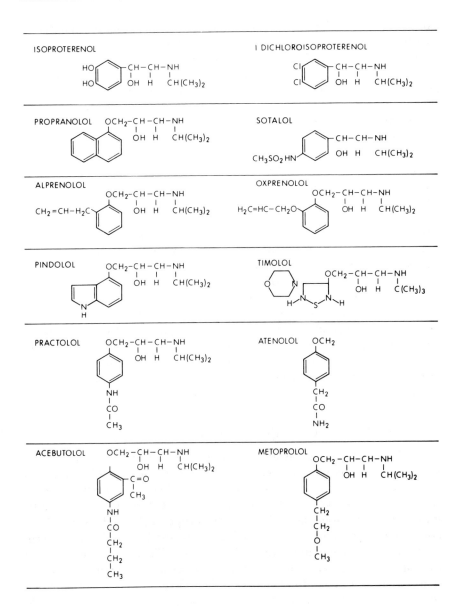

Figure 1-1. Structural formulas of available β-blocking drugs.

oxprenolol, pindolol, and practolol), cause a very small agonist response, indicating that they stimulate *and* block the receptor.[12] The partial agonist activity of these specific β-blocking drugs differs from that of epinephrine and isoproterenol, in that the maximum response which can be obtained is lower, although the affinity for the receptor site is high.[11]

On theoretical grounds, it may be postulated that β-blockers displaying ISA are less likely to induce cardiac insufficiency than β-blockers devoid of such activity, since the former will diminish the force of contraction of the heart muscle to a lesser extent.[21] Therapeutic studies have yet to demonstrate this supposition, however. It is of interest that β-blockers exhibiting no ISA, such as propranolol, cause an increase in pulmonary capillary wedge pressure and cardiopulmonary blood volume. Those drugs with ISA, such as oxprenolol and pindolol, either exert no influence on pulmonary capillary wedge pressure, or actually lower it, while at the same time, producing a smaller increase in cardiopulmonary blood volume.[22] β-Blockers which possess an intrinsic sympathomimetic effect lower the heart rate less markedly, and thus entail less risk of provoking excessive bradycardia.[23,24] A significant part of this excessive bradycardia results from unopposed, or enhanced, vagal activity, however, once the sympathetic tone has been inhibited.

There is no good evidence that β-blocking drugs with ISA are inherently safer in patients at risk from β-blockade (asthmatics) than those without ISA.[25] Pindolol, a drug with the most ISA among the β-blockers now in use, however, has been shown to be bronchoprotective in many patients intolerant to propranolol because of bronchospasm.[26]

CARDIOSELECTIVITY (TABLE 1-2)

β-Blockers may be classified as selective or nonselective. This is determined by their relative abilities to antagonize β-receptors in some tissues, at lower doses than are required for other tissues. When employed in low doses, cardioselective blockers inhibit the cardiac β-receptors (β_1) but exert little influence on the bronchial and vascular β-receptors (β_2).[27] Of the metabolic effects mediated by β-receptors, insulin release and liver and muscle glycogenolysis are mediated markedly by β_2-receptors. There is still doubt about the nature of the β-receptor mediating renin release and lipolysis. The fact that the cardioselective β-blocks have little or no effect on the peripheral β-receptors would, theoretically, have two advantages. First, these agents would be safe to employ in cases where the patient suffers or had suffered from bronchial asthma. Cardioselectivity is of undoubted therapeutic value. In clinical trials with asthmatic subjects, practolol caused a lower incidence of respiratory side effects than did propranolol.[28] However, other investigators have commented that some cardioselective β-blockers (i.e., practolol and acebutolol) may increase bronchial obstruction due to differences in asthmatic patients.[29] Second, β-blockers with cardioselectivity might appear suitable for the treatment of hypertension because their use would involve no inhibition of the peripheral (vasodilator) β-receptors.[23] In practice, however, cardioselectivity is diminished at the usual doses required for treatment of hypertension.[27]

In small doses, acebutolol, atenolol, metoprolol, and practolol ("cardioselective" blockers) are 50 to 100 times more active in inhibiting the effects of isoproterenol on heart rate and force of contraction (β_1-receptors), than on the smooth muscle of the bronchial tree and peripheral blood vessels (β_2-receptors).[11] The separation is evidently not absolute, and at higher doses, β_2 antagonism becomes apparent. Cardioselectivity is, therefore, dose-dependent and decreases or disappears when larger doses are used.[30] This is in sharp contrast to drugs having ISA. With higher doses, the ISA effect remains undiminished.

At this juncture, the exact basis for cardioselectivity is not understood.

DIFFERENCES IN PHARMACOKINETIC PROPERTIES (TABLES 1-3 AND 1-4)

The pharmacokinetics of propranolol have been studied more intensively than almost any other drug in the history of pharmacology. Soon after its introduction, its plasma concentration was demonstrated to be much lower and more variable after an oral, rather than an intravenous dose, although the drug was quickly and completely absorbed from the gastrointestinal tract.[31,32] This variance in bioavailability was also found with other β-blockers. In this section, the pharmacokinetic differences between these drugs will be discussed.

ABSORPTION

With the exception of atenolol, all the β-blocking compounds are well absorbed over a wide portion of the small intestine. Absorption is fairly rapid and peak blood concentrations occur 1 to 3 hours after administration. The absorption of "sustained release" preparations of alprenolol or oxprenolol is prolonged and lower peak blood levels are achieved.[11,32]

BIOAVAILABILITY OF ORALLY ADMINISTERED DRUGS

With drugs which are extensively metabolized by the liver, some of the administered dose fails to reach the circulation after oral administration, despite complete alimentary absorption. This is because the drug in the portal vein is taken up and removed by the liver before it can appear in the systemic circulation. Both propranolol and alprenolol undergo extensive obligatory presystemic hepatic ("first pass") elimination. In addition, the relationship between bioavailability and dose is not proportional, following oral administration of single doses. The availability of small doses is quite low.[11, 31] As the dose is increased, progressively more drug reaches the systemic circulation. These data suggest that the avid hepatic extraction pattern becomes saturated with larger doses.[12] This "first pass" effect may explain the wide variability in plasma concentrations seen in patients receiving the same dose of drug. This kinetic situation applies to the disposition of not only propranolol and alprenolol, but also to oxprenolol.[33]

One important consequence of the high first pass metabolism of propranolol is that an intravenous dose of the drug represents a much greater plasma concentration, in proportion to the oral dose, than would appear from the number of mg administered.

The bioavailability of other oral β-blocking agents is given in Table 1-3. Pindolol has somewhat different kinetics than propranolol and alprenolol, after both oral and intravenous administrations. It is unlikely that first pass metabolism is important here.[34] Practolol is the least extensively metabolized of the β-blockers, 90% being eliminated from the body unchanged (no first pass effect).[35]

LIPID SOLUBILITY AND PROTEIN BINDING (TABLE 1-3)

β-Blockers vary widely in their lipid solubility[31] and plasma protein-binding characteristics.[31, 32] Propranolol and alprenolol have the highest degree of lipid solubility.[31] This factor greatly influences the distribution volume of these drugs and may bear on their ability to cross the blood–brain barrier. Animal studies have shown that the highly lipid soluble drugs equilibrate rapidly between the brain and the plasma.[31] Practolol[36] and metoprolol[37] have a low degree of lipophilicity.

Binding to various protein fractions in the blood has a significant effect in the pharmacokinetic and pharmacodynamic properties of drugs. Generally, only the unbound fraction of the drug is considered effective when relating the pharmacologic effect to the plasma concentration. Only the free fraction of the drug should, therefore, be considered.[38] It is also generally appreciated that the degree of protein binding can have a pronounced effect on the elimination kinetics of drugs, particularly on those with high affinity for the proteins.

Binding of β-blockers to various serum proteins has been studied to a minor extent and the methods used in different investigations have varied. It is difficult to make relevant comparisons betwen reported results. It is

TABLE 1-3. Pharmacokinetic Parameters of β-Blockers[11,31]

Drug	Extent of absorption (% of dose)	Extent of bioavailability (% of dose)	Dose-dependent bioavailability	Variation in plasma level	Beta-blocking plasma conc.	Percent bound SERUM PROTEINS	Percent bound HSA*	Lipid solubility†
Acebutolol	—	—	—	—	0.2–2 μg/ml	—	—	—
Alprenolol	>90	≈10	Yes	10–20-fold	50–100 ng/ml	85	38	Strong
Atenolol	—	⩾40	No	low	0.2–0.5 μg/ml	—	—	Weak
Metoprolol	>95	≈50	No	7-fold	50–100 ng/ml	12	12	Strong
Oxprenolol	70–95	24–60	No	5-fold	80–100 ng/ml	—	—	Strong
Pindolol	>90	≈100	No	4-fold	50–150 ng/ml	—	57	Weak
Practolol	>95	≈100	No	—	1.5–5 μg/ml	—	32	Weak
Propranolol	>90	≈30	Yes	20-fold	50–100 ng/ml	93	62	Strong
Sotalol	—	⩾60	—	4-fold	0.5–4 μg/ml	—	54	—
Timolol	>90	—	—	—	?5–10 ng/ml	—	—	—

*HSA: Human serum albumin
†Lipid solubility determined by the distribution ratio between oxtanol and water.
From Waal-Manning HJ[11]; Johnsson, G, Regardh CG.[31]

quite obvious, however, that the degree of binding varies considerably between different compounds, despite structural relationships. Johansson et al.[39] found that serum protein binding of alprenolol is about 85 percent at therapeutic serum levels, whereas the binding of the less lipophilic metoprolol was only about 12 percent.[39]

VOLUME OF DISTRIBUTION, DRUG CLEARANCE, AND HALF LIFE (TABLE 1-4)

The β-blockers so far studied are rapidly distributed in the body. The apparent volume of distribution varies three to four-fold between the compounds but, in all cases, the apparent volume of distribution exceeds the physiologic body space.[31]

TABLE 1-4. **Elimination Characteristics of Some Orally Administered β-adrenoreceptor Blocking Drugs**

Drug	Elimination half-life (h)	Total body clearance (liters/min)	Urinary recovery of unchanged drug (% of dose)	Total urinary recovery (% of dose)	Active metabolites of clinical importance
Acebutolol	about 8	—	—	—	—
Alprenolol	2–3	1.2	<1	>90	Yes
Atenolol	6–9	—	≈40	—	No
Metoprolol	3–4	1.1	≈3	>95	No
Oxprenolol	2	0.6	—	70–95	—
Pindolol	3–4	0.4	≈40	>90	No
Practolol	6–8	0.14	>90	>90	No
Propranolol	3.5–6	1.0	<1	>90	Yes
Sotalol	5–13	—	≈60	—	—
Timolol	4–5	—	≈20	65	—

From Johnsson G, Regardh CG.[31]

The β-blockers are rapidly eliminated from the body. Most of them have an elimination half-life of between 2 to 4 hours. The shortest half-lives are found with those drugs that are extensively metabolized (practolol having the lowest rate of elimination). Even with respect to elimination, the various β-blockers show a diversified pattern that appears to be associated with the lipid solubility of the drug.[31] Highly fat soluble drugs, like alprenolol and propranolol, are almost completely eliminated by various metabolic systems in the liver.[31] As the lipid solubility decreases, renal excretion becomes more important. This mechanism appears to be almost entirely responsible for the elimination of practolol (low lipid solubility).[35] Between these extreme examples of the elimination pattern, there are several drugs for which both biotransformation and renal excretion significantly influence elimination (as shown by the ratio of unchanged drug and metabolites in the urine, see Table 1-4). The "urinary recovery of unchanged drug" in Table 1-4 refers to oral administration. It is important to note that for those compounds with a pronounced hepatic first pass elimination effect (alprenolol, propranolol), the fraction of the dose excreted unchanged in the urine will be substantially higher after intravenous administration.[31]

The mode of elimination of the different β-blocker compounds may have clinical relevance in patients with renal and hepatic disease. As practolol is mainly eliminated by the kidney, it can be expected that decreased renal function should have a pronounced effect on the pharmacokinetics of the drug. For practolol, a linear increase relationship between the plasma half-life and creatinine clearance has been obtained by a number of workers.[40,41] Bodem et al.[40] found an up to sixfold increase in plasma half life and, in uremic patients with a glomerular filtration rate below 3 ml per minute, plasma half-lives of over 100 hours have been recorded for practolol. During dialysis a considerable shortening of the half-life was found.[41]

Sotalol is also excreted primarily via the kidneys, as an unchanged drug. In patients with end-stage renal failure, the plasma half-life for sotalol was, on the average, 42 hours. This compared with 5 hours in normals.[42]

Despite its being 40 percent eliminated by the kidneys, the half-life of pindolol was not affected by renal disease, there being a concomitant increase in metabolic clearance as renal clearance was reduced.[43]

The effects of liver disease have not been investigated for β-blockers. For those drugs having a high hepatic clearance, a reduction in clearance and a prolonged half-life would be expected for several reasons, including reduced hepatic flow, decreased enzyme activity, and decreased protein binding.[32]

The variations in elimination rate of the β-blockers would appear to imply that therapy with these agents should be started at lower doses in patients with either liver disease (if the drug is mainly eliminated via metabolism in the liver) or renal disease (if the drug is mainly eliminated in unmetabolized form). It might be advisable to monitor plasma levels of the drugs in patients with liver or kidney disease.

RELATIONSHIP BETWEEN DOSE, PLASMA LEVEL, AND EFFICACY

β-Blockers that are largely metabolized by the liver show large interindividual variation in circulating drug concentrations, after a given oral dose. This is probably because of the first pass effect (alprenolol, propranolol) and genetic differences in the rate of drug metabolism (Table 1-3).[32] The variation is less for drugs largely cleared by renal mechanisms (practolol), provided that renal function is not impaired.

A wide variation also exists between plasma concentration of β-blockers and any associated therapeutic effect. There have been many explanations posed to explain this phenomenon. First, patients may have different levels of "sympathetic tone," therefore, a greater concentration of a given β-blocker would be required to achieve the desired therapeutic result. This was shown by our group with propranolol, where large differences in plasma drug levels were associated with the same pharmacologic effect.[44] Second, many β-blockers have flat plasma response curves. This means that the plasma concentration may vary considerably within a very narrow effect interval.[31]

Another reason may lie in the formation of varying amounts of active metabolites (not measured in plasma assay) in different individuals. This might be, for instance, the case with propranolol and alprenolol, both of which form active metabolites of clinical significance.[31,32]

Despite the lack of correlation between plasma levels and interpatient therapeutic effect, there is some evidence that a relationship does exist between the logarithm of the plasma level and the β-blocking effect (blockade of exercise-induced tachycardia or isoproterenol-induced tachycardia).[31] The β-blocking plasma concentrations for the different compounds are shown in Table 1-3.

Several authors have reported that the duration of the β-blocking effect is considerably longer than indicated by the elimination half lives of the β-blockers.[31,35] A pronounced decrease in the plasma concentration with time may, therefore, not be associated with a parallel decrement in clinical effect. This has been demonstrated in clinical practice where, it has been shown that many of the β-blocker compounds can be administered once or twice daily.[31]

CONCLUSION

Although β-blocking compounds have similar therapeutic effects, they have different pharmacologic properties. Understanding these differences may enable the clinician to select a specific compound for a given clinical situation.

REFERENCES

1. Ahlquist RP: A study of the adrenotropic receptors. Am J Physiol 153:586–599, 1948
2. Lands AM, Arnold A, McAuliff JP, Luduena FP, Brown TG: Differentiation of receptor systems activated by sympathomimetic amines. Nature 214:597–598, 1967

3. Dunlop D, Shanks RG: Selective blockade of adrenoceptive beta-receptors in the heart. Br J Pharmacol 32:201-218, 1968
4. Lefkowitz RJ: Selectivity in beta-adrenergic response. Circulation 49:783-785, 1974
5. Powell CE, Slater IH: Blocking of inhibitory adrenergic receptors by a dichloro-analog of isoproterenol. J Pharmacol Exp Ther 122:480-488, 1958
6. Black JW, Stephenson JS: Pharmacology of a new adrenergic beta-receptor blocking compound (nethalide). Lancet 2:311-314, 1962
7. Status report on beta blockers. FDA Drug Bulletin 8:13, 1978
8. Wright P: Untoward effect associated with practolol administration oculomucocutaneous syndrome. Br Med J 1:595-598, 1975
9. Windsor WP, Durrein F, Dyer NH: Fibrinous peritonitis: A complication of practolol therapy. Br Med J 2:68, 1975
10. Dollery CT, Paterson JW, Connolly MI: Clinical pharmacology of beta receptor blocking drugs. Clin Pharmacol Ther 10:765-799, 1969
11. Waal-Manning HJ: Hypertension: which beta-blocker? Drugs 12:412-441, 1976
12. Connolly ME, Keusting F, Dollery CT: The clinical pharmacology of beta-adrenoceptor blocking drug. Prog Cardiovasc Dis 19:203-234, 1976
13. Goodman LS, Gilman A: The Pharmacological Basis of Therapeutics. London, Collier,MacMillan 1970, pp 484-487, 566
14. Barrett AM, Cullum VA: The biological properties of the optical isomers of propranolol and their effects on cardiac arrhythmias. Br J Pharmacol 34:43-55, 1968
15. Åblad B, Brugård M, Ek L: Pharmacologic properties of H 56/28, a beta adrenergic receptor antagonist. Acta Pharmacol Toxicol 25 (Supp. 2): 9-40, 1967
16. Brunner H, Hedwall PR, Maier R et al.: Pharmacological aspects of oxprenolol. Postgrad Med J 46 (Nov. suppl):5-14, 1970
17. Basil B, Jordan R, Loveless AH, et al.: b-adrenoceptor blocking properties and cardioselectivity of M and B 17, 803 A. Br J Pharmacol 48:198-211, 1973
18. Singh BN: Clinical aspects of the anti-arrhythmic action of beta-receptor blocking drugs. Part 2. Clinical pharmacology. NZ Med J 78:529-535, 1973
19. Coltart OJ, Gibson DG, Shand DG: Plasma propranolol levels associated with suppressing of ectopic bouts. Br Med J I:490-491, 1971
20. Singh BN, Jewitt DE: B-adrenergic receptor clocking drugs in cardiac arrhythmias. Drugs 7:426-461, 1974
21. Choquet Y, Capone RJ, Mason DT, Amsterdam EA, Zelis R: Comparison of the beta adrenergic blocking properties and negative inotropic effects of oxprenolol and propranolol in patients. Am J Cardio 29:257, 1972 (abstract)
22. Majid PA, Saxton C, Stoker JB, Taylor SH: Comparison of the hemodynamic effects of acute intravenous and oral therapy with proproanolol and oxprenolol in hypertensive patients. Cardiovasc. Res. 6. London, VIth World Congress Cardiology, 1970, p. 208
23. Imhof PR: Characterization of beta blockers as anti-hypertensive agents in the light of human pharmocology studies. In Schweizer W (ed): Beta-Blockers — Present Status and Future Prospects. Bern, Huber, 1974, pp. 40-50
24. Frishman W, Kostis J, Strom J, et al.: Clinical pharmacology of the new beta-adrenergic blocking drugs. Part 6. A comparison of pindolol and propranolol in treatment of patients with angina pectoris. The role of intrinsic sympathomimetic activity. Am Heart J 98: 526, 1979.

25. Addis GJ, Thorp JM: Effects of oxprenolol on the airways of normal and bronchitic subjects. Eur J Clin Pharmacol 9: 259-263, 1976

26. Frishman W, Davis R, Strom J, et al.: Clinical pharmacology of the beta-adrenergic blocking drugs. Part 5. Pindolol (LB-46) therapy for supraventricular arrhythmia: A viable alternative to propranolol in patients with bronchospasm. Am Heart J 98: 393, 1979

27. Fitzgerald JD: Cardioselective beta adrenergic blockage Proc Royal Soc Med 65: 761-764, 1972

28. MacDonald AG, McNeill RS: A comparison of the effect on airway resistance of a new beta blocking drug ICI 50, 172 and propranolol. Br J Anaesthesiol 40: 508-510, 1968

29. Skinner C, Palmer KNV, Kerridge DF: Comparison of the effects of acebutolol (Sectral) and practolol on airways obstruction in asthmatics. Br J Clin Pharmacol 2: 417-422, 1975

30. Lertora JJL, Mark AL, Johannsen UJ, Wilson WR, Abboud FM: Selective beta-1 receptor blockade with oral practolol in man. J Clin Invest 56: 719-724, 1975

31. Johnsson G, Regardh CG: Clinical pharmacokinetics of b-adrenoreceptors blocking drugs. Clin Pharmacokin I: 233-263, 1976

32. Shand DG: Pharmacokinetic properties of the b-adrenergic receptor blocking drugs. Drugs 7: 39-47, 1974

33. Riess W, Huerzeler H, Ruschdorf F: The metabolites of oxprenolol (Trasicor) in man. Xenobiotica 4:365-373, 1974

34. Gugler R, Herold W, Dengler HJ: Pharmacokinetics of pindolol in man. Eur J Clin Pharmacol 17:24, 1974

35. Carruthers SG, Kelly JG, McDevitt DG, Shanks RG: Blood levels of practolol and oral and parenteral administration and their relationship to exercise heart rate. Clin Pharmacol Ther 15: 497-509, 1974

36. Bodin NO, Borg KO, Johansson R, Ramsay CH, Skanberg I: The distribution of metoprolol-(^{3}H) in the mouse and rat. Acta Pharmacol Toxicol 36 (Suppl. V):116-124, 1975

37. Scales B, Cosgrove MD: The metabolism and distribution of the selective adrenergic beta blocking agent practolol. J Pharmacol Exper Ther 175: 338-347, 1970

38. Koch-Weser J, Sellers EM: Binding of drugs to serum albumin (second of two parts) N Eng J Med 294: 526-531, 1976

39. Johansson KA, Appelgren C, Borg KO, Elofsson R: Binding of two adrenergic beta-receptor antagonists, alprenolol and H 93/26 to human serum proteins. Acta Pharmacol Suecica 8: 59-70, 1971

40. Bodem G, Greiser H, Eichelbaum M, Gugler R: Pharmacokinetics of practolol in renal failure. Eur J Clin Pharm 7: 249-252, 1974

41. Eastwood JB, Curtis JR, Smith RB: Pharmacodynamics of practolol in chronic renal failure. Br Med J 4: 320-322, 1973

42. Tjandramaga TB, Thomas J, Verbeeck R, et al.: The effect on end-stage renal failure and hemodialysis on the elimination kinetics of sotalol. Br J Clin Pharmacol 3: 259-265, 1975

43. Ohnhaus EE, Neusch E, Meier J, Kalbarer F: Pharmacokinetics of labelled and ^{14}C-unlabelled pindolol in uraemia. Eur J Clin Pharmacol 7: 25-29, 1974

44. Frishman W, Smithen C, Befler B, Kligfield P, Killip T: Non-invasive assessment of clinical response to oral propranolol. Am J Cardiol 35: 635-644, 1975

CHAPTER TWO

Physiologic and Metabolic Effects

William H. Frishman and Ralph Silverman

TWO decades after their discovery, the therapeutic use of β-adrenoceptor blocking drugs has been well established in angina pectoris, cardiac arrhythmias, and hypertension. β-Blockers are also being used for a growing number of new indications.

Some of the basic pharmacodynamic and pharmacokinetic differences between β-blocking agents have been discussed in the previous chapter. The main emphasis of this chapter is directed toward their physiologic and metabolic effects in man.

CARDIOVASCULAR EFFECTS

EFFECTS IN HYPERTENSION (Table 2-1 and 2-2):

It is now well recognized that β-adrenergic blockers are effective in controlling the blood pressure of many patients with hypertension. At the present time, there is no consensus of opinion as to the mechanism(s) whereby these drugs lower blood pressure. It is probable that some or all of the following play a part.

1. Negative Chronotropic and Inotropic Effects. Slowing of the heart rate and some decrease in myocardial contractility lead to a decrease in cardiac output, which, in the long term, may lead to a reduction in blood pressure.[1] It might be expected that this factor would be of particular importance in treatment of hypertension related to high cardiac output.[2]

2. A Central Nervous System Effect. There is good clinical and experimental evidence that β-blockers enter the central nervous system.[3] The occurrence of dreams, insomnia, hallucinations, and depression during ther apy with β-blockers supports this conjecture.

Infusion of L and DL-propranolol into the cerebral ventricles of conscious rabbits caused a marked antihypertensive effect, whereas D-propranolol caused the blood pressure to rise.[4] By injecting drugs into the vertebral arteries of anesthetized dogs, other investigators found a central antihypertensive action for alprenolol but not for propranolol.[5] Although there is little doubt that β-blockers (especially those with high lipophilicity, e.g., alprenolol, propranolol) enter the central nervous system in high concentrations, an antihypertensive effect mediated by their presence is not as yet well defined.

3. Differences in Effects on Plasma Renin. The relationship between the hypotensive action of β-blocking drugs and their ability to reduce plasma renin activity is currently one of the more hotly disputed areas in the field of hypertension. There is no doubt that β-blocking drugs can antagonize sympathetically mediated renin release.[6] Adrenergic activity is not the only mechanism whereby renin release is mediated, however. Other major determinants are sodium balance, posture, and renal perfusion pressure.

Laragh[6] and his group have suggested that a decrease in renin output by the kidney is the major factor in the antihypertensive effect of β-blockers. Propranolol lowers plasma renin activity in normal[7] and hypertensive subjects[8] and blocks the orthostatic rise in plasma renin activity on standing.[9] Dextro propranolol has no effect on renin release, which is inhibited by racemic propranolol in the same patients,[9] and has no effect on plasma renin activity in the rabbit.[10] The suppressant effect of racemic propranolol is therefore dependent on the β-blocking action of the levoisomers.

The effect of the different β-blockers on resting and orthostatic renin release is variable. Among the nonselective blockers: propranolol causes the greatest reduction of both resting and orthostatic renin release,[11] timolol causes significant reduction,[12] oxprenolol,[13] and alprenolol[14] have less effect (especially on orthostatic renin release); and pindolol has the least effect. Weber et al.[10] found that, in the rabbit, pindolol causes a rise in plasma renin activity; Stokes et al.[15] found that patients switched from propranolol to pindolol continued to have good control of their blood pressure despite a rise in plasma renin activity.[10] It has been suggested that the smaller effect of alprenolol, oxprenolol, and pindolol on renin, compared with propranolol, may be due to their partial agonist properties.[15]

The cardioselective β-blockers show similar variation in effect; practolol has no effect on renin[16]; metoprolol lowers resting and furosemide-induced renin release[17,18]; atenolol has conflicting reports. (Amery et al.[19] showed no effect, whereas Aberg[20] demonstrated a significant decrease in resting renin.) The lack of a renin-lowering effect with practolol may be related to its partial agonist activity. The effectiveness of the other two cardioselective β-blockers may suggest that, at least in man, renin release is mediated by a β_1-receptor. But other studies in experimental animal propose a β_2-receptor for renin release[10] and the question remains a matter of controversy.

The crucial question, however, is whether there is a clinical correlation between the β-blocker effect on plasma renin activity and the lowering of blood pressure. Laragh's group[6] found that "high-renin" patients respond well to propranolol, "low-renin" patients do not respond or may even show a rise in blood pressure, and "normal renin" patients have less predictable responses.

Using alprenolol, Castenfors[13] found a correlation between fall in plasma renin activity and fall in blood pressure. Other authors have been unable to confirm this relationship, however, either for propranolol or for other β-blockers.[15,21] Even in the "high-renin" hypertensive, it has been suggested that renin may not be the only factor maintaining the high blood pressure. At present, the exact roles of renin and β-blockade in blood pressure control are not defined.

4. Venous Tone. Reduced plasma volume and venous return may play a role in the control of blood pressure by β-blockers. A few studies have shown these effects, "in both acute and long" term therapy, when heart failure was not present.[22] Since one would expect an impaired cardiac output to cause an increase in plasma volume, these early findings, though not yet fully investigated, are of great interest.

5. Peripheral Resistance. β-blockade has no primary action in lowering peripheral resistance and, indeed, may cause it to rise by unopposed α stimulation.[23] The vasodilating effect of catecholamines on skeletal muscle blood vessels is β_2-mediated, suggesting a possible advantage of cardiospecific β_1-blockers or drugs with partial agonist effects in therapy. Since cardioselectivity diminishes as the dosage is raised, however, and since hypertensive patients generally have to be given far larger doses than are required simply to block the β_1-receptors, this cardioselectivity[24] is only relative and offers little if any real advantage.

6. "Quinidine Effect" (Membrane Stabilizing). Some early investigative studies[25] indicated that the antihypertensive effect of propranolol paralleled the antihypertensive effect of quinidine, suggesting that the "membrane-stabilizing" effect might be important. Later studies refuted these early findings, however.[26] All the β-blockers appear to reduce blood pressure, regardless of the presence of "membrane" effects.[18] This has been confirmed since D-propranolol, with predominant "membrane" effects, does not affect blood pressure.

In summary, β-blockers have been found to be useful in hypertension, although their precise mechanism of action remains unclear. Whether cardioselective β-blockers or agents with partial agonist activity will prove more or less advantageous as compared with nonselective β-blocking drugs, has yet to be determined.

ANGINA PECTORIS: EFFECTS ON HEART RATE AND MYOCARDIAL CONTRACTILITY (TABLE 2-1)

In 1948 Ahlquist[27] demonstrated that sympathetic innervation of the heart causes the release of norepinephrine which activates β-adrenoreceptors in myocardial cells. The effects of this stimulation cause an increase in heart rate, isometric force, and maximal velocity of muscle fiber shortening, leading to an increase in cardiac work and myocardial oxygen consumption.[28] The decrease in intraventricular pressure and volume, caused by the sympathetic mediated enhancement of cardiac contractility, tends, on the other hand, to reduce myocardial oxygen consumption by reducing myocardial wall tension (Law of LaPlace).[29] Although there is a net increase in myocardial oxygen demand, this is normally balanced by an increase in coronary blood flow. Angina pectoris is felt to occur when oxygen demand exceeds supply, i.e., when coronary blood flow is restricted by coronary atherosclerosis. Since the conditions which precipitate anginal attacks (exercise, emotional stress, food, etc.) cause an increase in cardiac sympathetic activity, it might be expected that blockade of cardiac β-adrenoreceptors would relieve the symptoms of the anginal syndrome. It is on this basis that the initial clinical studies of β-blocking drugs in angina were initiated.[30] These studies led to the development of one of the most important therapeutic discoveries of the past two decades.

Four main factors — heart rate, ventricular systolic pressure, rate of rise of left ventricular pressure, and the size of the left ventricle — contribute to the oxygen demand of the left ventricle. Of these, heart rate and systolic pressure appear to be the most important (heart rate times systolic blood pressure product is a reliable index to predict the precipitation of angina in a given patient).[31]

The reduction of heart rate effected by β-blockade has two important beneficial effects: (1) Decrease in cardiac work, thereby reducing oxygen demand, and (2) the longer diastolic filling time associated with slower heart rate allows for greater coronary perfusion time. β-blockade also reduces exercise-induced blood pressure rise, velocity of cardiac contraction, and oxygen consumption at any workload.[32]

Studies in dogs have shown propranolol causes a decrease in coronary blood flow.[33] However, subsequent work in dogs demonstrated shunting within the coronary circulation with β-blockade in a manner that maintains blood flow to ischemic areas, especially in the subendocardial region.[34] In man, simultaneous with the decrease in myocardial oxygen consumption, β-blockade also causes a reduction in coronary blood flow and a rise in coronary vascular resistance.[32] The overall decrease in oxygen consumption by the heart as a whole may be sufficient cause for the decrease in coronary blood flow, however.

Virtually all β-blockers whether or not they have partial agonist activity, membrane-stabilizing activity, general or selective β-blocking properties, produce some degree of increased work capacity without pain. Therefore, it must be concluded that this results from their common characteristic: blockade of cardiac β-receptors.[35] For example, both D- and L-propranolol have membrane-stabilizing activity but only L-propranolol has significant β-blocking activity. The racemic mixture (D- and L-propranolol) causes a decrease in heart rate and force of contraction in dogs, while the D-isomer has hardly any effect.[36] In man, D-propranolol, which has "membrane" but no β-blocking properties has been found ineffective in angina pectoris using very high doses.[37]

The effect of β-blocking drugs in acute exercise versus angina pectoris is of interest. Although exercise tolerance improves (the increment in heart rate and blood pressure with exercise is blunted), the pressure rate product (systolic blood pressure times heart rate) achieved when pain occurs is less than that reached during a control run.[38] This depressed pressure-rate product at the onset of pain (about 20 percent reduction from control) occurred with various intravenously administered β-blocking drugs that differed in certain properties: propranolol (membrane-stabilizing activity), oxprenolol (membrane-stabilizing and intrinsic sympathomimetic activity), practolol (cardioselective blockade and intrinsic sympathomimetic activity), and sotalol (minimal membrane-stabilizing activity).[39] Thus, although there is increased exercise tolerance with β-blockade, patients exercise less than might be expected. This probably represents the potentially adverse effect of β-blockers in increasing left ventricular size, causing increased left ventricular wall tension and an increase in oxygen consumption at a given blood pressure.[40]

All β-blockers will limit the heart rate increment with exercise; however, they cause differing effects on the resting heart rate. Propranolol and metoprolol slow the resting pulse more than do oxprenolol, pindolol, and practolol; D-propranolol had very little resting pulse slowing activity. Morgan et al.[41] also found differences in pulse slowing activity among four β-blockers they tested: propranolol and timolol reduced pulse rate more than pindolol and alprenolol. It would appear that β-blockers lacking partial agonist activity slow the resting pulse rate more than the β-blockers that have partial agonist activity.

A possible explanation as to why drugs with intrinsic sympathomimetic activity do not affect the resting heart rate to the same degree as they affect the increment in heart rate with exercise is probably related to the increased sympathetic tone with exercise. At rest, without a high degree of sympathetic activity, the intrinsic sympathomimetic effect will be more apparent than the β-blocking effect, the converse being true with exercise.

The therapeutic benefit of β-blockade in angina pectoris is now established beyond question. There are many double blind studies demonstrating a significant lowering in the frequency of anginal attacks. Observed improvement is dose-related and dosage must be titrated for each individual patient. All the various β-blockers, despite their differing characteristics and activities, have some effect in the relief of angina.

Propranolol is the most widely used β-blocker today. It is nonselective, has membrane-stabilizing activity, but has no intrinsic sympathomimetic activity. There have been numerous trials of propranolol, using fixed single and multiple dose level trials, that have shown its efficacy in angina pectoris in a dose-related manner.[42] Alprenolol and oxprenolol, which appeared soon after propranolol was introduced, are, like propranolol, nonselective β-blockers with membrane-stabilizing activity and good antianginal effects. Unlike propranolol, they both possess intrinsic sympathomimetic activity. Although trial studies for the most part have shown beneficial effects from both drugs, the presence or absence of a dose–response relationship for alprenolol has not been firmly established.

Sotalol is a nonselective β-blocker, with neither intrinsic sympathomimetic activity nor any membrane-stabilizing activity. In an acute intravenous study, Prichard[43] found it equivalent to propranolol and minimally superior to oxprenolol in delaying the onset of pain. In a longer oral dose study, however, Horn and Prichard[44] found propranolol to be more effective. Other studies[45,46] have shown the two drugs to be roughly equivalent. Timolol, another nonselective β-blocker with neither intrinsic sympathomimetic activity nor "membrane effect," was shown in a large multicenter trial to be effective in reducing the frequency of anginal attacks.[47]

Nonselective β-blockers are contraindicated in patients with obstructive airway disease. The development of selective β_1-blockers, therefore, has had important therapeutic implications (although cardioselectivity is not absolute and decreases with increasing dose). Practolol, which has intrinsic sympathomimetic activity and cardioselectivity, was the first of these agents and, while in use, was found to be effective, though less so than propranolol in equivalent doses.[43] However, with increased reports of serious toxic effects (SLE-type syndrome, eye lesions, skin lesions, sclerosing peritonitis), the drug was withdrawn. Recently, other cardioselective β-blockers have been developed.

Atenolol differs from practolol in that it lacks intrinsic sympathomimetic activity. In an acute study comparing atenolol with propranolol in severe angina, both drugs produced an equal reduction in exercise-induced tachycardia, but atenolol produced a higher maximal working capacity than propranolol.[48] This increased work capacity may reflect the lack of interference by atenolol on the peripheral vascular adaptation to exercise. Roy,[49] in comparing atenolol with placebo, found that it significantly reduced the number of nitroglycerin tablets consumed and the frequency of angina attacks.

Metoprolol is another selective β-blocker devoid of intrinsic sympathomimetic activity whose preliminary data indicate its effectiveness in angina.[41]

In summary, all β-blockers, despite their differing pharmocodynamic properties, are effective in angina pectoris, blunting the heart rate-blood pressure-contractility increments in exercise. This enables patients to do more work at lower oxygen demands, despite increments in end-diastolic volume, and myocardial wall tension. Whether or not drugs with intrinsic sympathomimetic activity (e.g., pindolol) will prove safer than propranolol due to the potential lessening of myocardial depression is yet to be determined.

ARRHYTHMIAS (TABLE 2-1)

Although β-blocking drugs have been used for treating cardiac arrhythmias for over a decade, their precise mode of action remains unclear. Two main effects of these drugs, β-blockade and membrane-stabilizing activity, have been identified:

1. β-Blockade. By blocking adrenergic stimulation of cardiac pacemaker potentials, β-blocking drugs are useful in controlling arrhythmias that are caused by enhanced automaticity and reentry. In concentrations which cause significant inhibition of cardiac adrenergic receptors, the slope of the pacemaker action potential (either sinus or ectopic) is reduced, particularly in the presence of catecholamines or ouabain.[50,51] Thus, arrhythmias related to sympathetic hyperactivity would be expected to respond to β-blockade. Similarly, in myocardial infarction, where there is increased levels of circulating catecholamines causing enhanced automaticity, β-blockers are likely to be useful.[52] This is not to say, however, that β-blockers will *only* be effective in arrhythmias directly related to catecholamines (e.g., pheochromocytoma, halothane anesthesia). Clinically, their usefulness has been demonstrated in many other types of arrhythmias as well. Their beneficial effect in these situations probably derives from removal of normal adrenergic effects that may be unfavorably additive to the major arrhythmias-causing stimulus. One such example would be arrhythmias related to digitalis toxicity.[53]

2. Membrane-Stabilizing Action. The second possible mechanism explaining the antiarrhythmic effect of β-blocking drugs is their membrane-stabilizing or depressing action, often referred to as the "quinidinelike" or

TABLE 2–1. Pharmacodynamic Properties and Cardiac Effects of β-Adrenoceptor Drugs

Drug	Cardio-selectivity*	Partial agonist activity	Membrane stabilizing activity	Resting heart rate	Rate of heart rate increment in response to exercise	Myocardial contractility	Resting blood pressure	Resting atrioventricular conduction	Antiarrhythmic effect
Acebutolol	+	+	+	↓	↓	↓	↓	↓	+
Alprenolol	0	++	+	↕	↓	↕	↓	↕	++
Atenolol	+	0	0	↓	↓	↓	↓	↓	++
Metoprolol	+	0	±	↕	↓	↓	↓	↕	++
Oxprenolol	0	++	+	↕	↓	↕	↓	↕	++
Pindolol	0	+++	0	↕	↓	↕	↓	↓	++
Practolol	+	++	0	↓	↓	↓	↓	↓	++
Propranolol	0	0	++	↓	↓	↓	↓	↓	++
Sotalol	0	0	0	↓	↓	↓	↓	↓	++
Timolol	0	±	0	↓	↓	↓	↓	↓	++
Isomer:									
D-Propranolol	0	0	++	↔	↕	↔↓†	↕	↔↓†	+–†

*Cardioselectivity of certain β-blockers is only seen with low therapeutic concentrations of drugs. With higher concentrations cardioselectivity is not seen.

†Effects of D-propranolol occur with doses in humans well above the therapeutic level. The isomer also lacks β-blocking activity.

"local anesthetic" action. This property is unrelated to inhibition of the action of catecholamines, and is held to an equal extent by both the D- and L-isomers of the drugs (D-isomers have virtually no β-blocking activity).[54] It is characterized by a reduction in the rate of rise of the intracardiac action potential without effecting the duration of the spike or the resting potential.[55] The effect has been explained by an inhibition of the depolarizing inward sodium current.

It should be noted, however, that in in vitro experiments with human ventricular muscle, the concentration of propranolol required to produce this effect is 50 to 100 times the concentration generally associated with inhibition of exercise-induced tachycardia.[56] The concentrations of propranolol needed to produce this effect are in the *milli*molar range, whereas general clinically used doses produce *micro*molar concentrations, at which level only β-blocking effects occur.

It seems probable, therefore, that in usual therapeutic doses, the main factor in the antiarrhythmic effect of these drugs is β-blockade. Coltart et al.[57] and Shand[58] have shown that arrhythmias are suppressed by plasma propranolol concentrations 1/50th to 1/100th of the level needed for membrane-stabilizing action. Jewitt and Singh[59] have observed that D-propranolol, which possesses membrane-stabilizing properties but no β-blocking action is weak as an antiarrhythmic even in very high doses. Practolol, on the other hand, is clinically effective as an antiarrhythmic, although it lacks membrane-stabilizing characteristics.

If β-blockade is, indeed, the major mechanism for antiarrhythmic effect, and the clinical relevance of membrane-stabilizing properties is negligible, then we would expect all β-blockers to have similar antiarrhythmic effects for a comparable degree of β-blockade. This, in fact, appears to be the case. No superiority of one β-blocking agent over another in the treatment of arrhythmias has yet been demonstrated. Any differences in their overall clinical effects must, therefore, be assumed to be related to their other associated pharmocologic properties.[60]

EFFECTS ON THE SINUS NODE AND ATRIOVENTRICULAR CONDUCTION

In animals and in man, β-blockers slow the rate of discharge of the sinus and ectopic pacemakers and increase the functional refractory period of the *atrioventricular* (AV) node. They also slow both antegrade and retrograde conduction in anomalous pathways.[61]

Since all β-blockers studied so far cause an increase in atrioventricular conduction time, advancing AV block is a potential complication when β-blockers are used in managing arrhythmias. From both animal and human studies, it is apparent that those β-blockers like propranolol, which do not

possess intrinsic sympathomimetic activity but have potent membrane-stabilizing properties, cause the greatest increase in atrioventricular conduction time. In contrast, Giudicelli et al.[62] showed that the partial agonist activity (intrinsic sympathomimetic activity) of pindolol, practolol, and alprenolol provides protection from the AV conduction impairment induced
by β-blockade.

It should also be noted that β-blocking drugs can, in large doses, induce
sinus node dysfunction that may lead to sinus arrest or sinoatrial block. β-
blocking drugs, therefore, are best avoided in patients with "sick sinus syndrome," which could be aggravated by β-blockade.

VASCULAR RESISTANCE AND PERIPHERAL BLOOD FLOW (TABLE 2-2)

Isoproterenol mediates its effects on cardiac contractility through the
β_1-receptor and its peripheral vasodilatory effects through the β_2-receptor.
Propranolol, by blocking both receptors, leaves uninhibited the α-adrener-
gic tone in the periphery. This would tend to increase peripheral vascular
resistance, an effect which has been clearly demonstrated with
propranolol.[63] This increase in peripheral resistance might potentiate the
rate-lowering effect of propranolol and negate some of its antihypertensive
properties.[24] This increase in peripheral resistance can affect blood flow in
the limbs, coronary arteries,[32] renal circulation,[64] splanchnic vessels,[65] and in
the brain.[66] Drugs with β_1-cardioselectivity (e.g., practolol) have little or no
effect on peripheral vessels (in doses where the drugs are cardioselective)
and tend therefore not to increase peripheral resistance.[24] Drugs with intrinsic sympathomimetic activity (e.g., pindolol) do not raise peripheral resistance as much as propranolol.[24]

Inhibition of peripheral vasodilation probably is the mechanism of the
beneficial effect of propranolol in migraine.[67] Pindolol and alprenolol, perhaps because of their partial agonist activity, have shown little or no effect in
the treatment of patients with migraine.

NONCARDIOVASCULAR EFFECTS

OXYGEN TRANSPORT (EFFECTS ON THE OXYHEMOGLOBIN DISSOCIATION CURVE)

Altered oxyhemoglobin dissociation could facilitate oxygen availability to poorly perfused zones of myocardium in patients with ischemic heart
disease.

It was suggested that the oxyhemoglobin dissociation curve could be
affected by administration of β-blocking drugs. Oski and Miller[68] showed
that propranolol produced a favorable alteration of the curve to the right in

TABLE 2–2.   Pharmacodynamic Properties and Some Noncardiac Effects of β-Adrenoceptor Drugs

Drug	Cardio-selectivity*	Partial agonist activity	Membrane stabilizing activity	Bronchoconstriction	Platelet aggregability	Plasma renin activity	Peripheral Resistance
Acebutolol	+	+	+	↑↓		↓↑	↑↓
Alprenolol	0	++	+	↑↓		↓↑	↑↓
Atenolol	+	0	0	↑↓		↓↑	↑↓
Metoprolol	+	0	±	↑↓		↓↑	↑↓
Oxprenolol	0	++	+	↑↓		↓↑	↑↓
Pindolol	0	+++	+	↑↓	→	↓↑	→↑↓
Practolol	+	++	0	↑↓	→	↓↑	↑↓
Propranolol	0	0	++	↑↓	↓↑	→	←
Sotalol	0	0	0	↑↓	→	→	←
Timolol	0	0	0	↑↓		→	←

*Cardioselectivity of certain β-blockers is only seen with low therapeutic concentrations of drugs. With higher concentrations cardioselectivity is not seen.

normal subjects, probably by a release of membrane bound 2,3 diphospho-glycerate (2,3 DPG). These results were not confirmed by Brain, who found no significant change in P_{50} (PO_2 at 50 percent hemoglobin saturation) using a higher oral dose of propranolol, and no alteration in erythrocyte 2,3 DPG.[69] We, also, were not able to corroborate the findings of Oski regarding changes in P_{50} and 2,3 DPG (during rest and with exercise) in patients with angina pectoris treated with propranolol or pindolol.[70-72].

Although other β-blockers have not yet been well investigated, it seems that the effects of β-blockers on the oxygen dissociation curve and on O_2 delivery are negligible.

EFFECTS ON THE BRONCHIAL TREE (TABLE 2-2)

Bronchodilation is mediated through catecholamine stimulation of the β_2-receptors in the lung. Propranolol, which blocks β-receptors (β_1 and β_2) can precipitate bronchospasm in some patients.

All β-blocking drugs, including those with cardioselectivity and partial agonist activity, can induce bronchoconstriction in patients with asthma and bronchitis. Comparative studies have shown, however, that compounds with partial agonist activity (alprenolol, pindolol, practolol)[73,74] and cardioselectivity (practolol, metoprolol)[75,76] are less likely to increase airway resistance (as measured by forced expiratory volume in one second [FEV_1]) in asthmatics than propranolol. Nevertheless, practolol[77] despite cardioselectivity and partial agonist activity, can induce bronchospasm in susceptible individuals.[77] Patients who develop asthma while taking a cardioselective β-blocker will respond readily with bronchodilation from standard doses of β_2-stimulant drugs such as salbutamol, whereas patients taking a nonselective β-blocker like propranolol will not.[78]

EFFECTS OF β-ADRENERGIC BLOCKING AGENTS ON METABOLISM

Hypoglycemia has been reported as a side effect of nonselective β-blockade in diabetics on insulin.[79] The severity of this insulin-induced hypoglycemia may be lessened with cardioselective β-blockers.[80,81] The symptoms of hypoglycemia are also modified by propranolol but sweating is enhanced.[82,83]

In man, epinephrine stimulates glycolysis in skeletal muscle predominantly via β-adrenoceptors, and in the liver predominantly via α-adrenoceptors.[84] In normal subjects, abolition of glucose mobilization requires simultaneous blockade of α-adrenergic receptors in the liver and β-adrenergic receptors in skeletal muscle, with phenoxybenzamine and propranolol, respectively.[85] Resting plasma glucose and insulin concentrations in normal individuals are not affected by propranolol. The fall of plasma glucose levels after administration of insulin is also unaffected. The rate of return of blood glucose levels to normal, however, after insulin-induced hypoglycemia, is reduced and the increase of plasma glycerol in prevented. These effects depend, in part, on the β-adrenergic effect of catecholamines reflexly released in response to the hypoglycemia. For this reason, in diabetics treated with insulin, and in some other situations (e.g., fasting), β-blockade with propranolol may be associated with hypoglycemia.[86]

In contrast, propranolol has been reported to precipitate hyperglycemia and hyperosmolar nonketotic coma, and to prevent recurrent hypoglycemia in a patient with insulinoma.[87,88]

These contrasting effects result from an interplay of several factors: gluconeogenesis, liver and skeletal muscle glycogenolysis, peripheral glucose utilization, and growth hormone, glucagon, and insulin secretion. β-Blockers inhibit glucose-sulfonylurea-stimulated insulin secretion. There is good evidence that the β-receptor for insulin secretion is of the β_2 type.[89]

Administration of propranolol has been shown to reduce plasma free fatty acid levels at rest, after prolonged fasting and during exercise, emotion, or insulin-induced hypoglycemia.[90,91] Also, propranolol, but not practolol, blocks the lipolytic activity of isoproterenol.[92,93] The increase in free fatty acids occurring during epinephrine infusion is blocked by propranolol, but accentuated by phentolamine, suggesting the presence of an additional inhibitory α-adrenergic mechanism.[94] The lipolytic activity of epinephrine can also be blocked by practolol, but only at doses significantly higher than those affecting its cardiovascular manifestations.[95] Thus, although the receptor sites associated with adrenergic stimulation of lipolysis fulfill many of the characteristics of a β-receptor, the presence of an inhibitory effect that can be reversed by phentolamine, and a reduced sensitivity to practolol, show that they are not identical with those affecting heart rate and force of contraction.

Although the metabolic effects of β-blockade are not nearly as prominent as their hemodynamic effects, and the incidence of metabolic side effects is low, β-adrenergic-blocking agents should be used with caution in patients prone to hypoglycemia, particularly insulin-treated diabetics. Cardioselective blockers, (e.g., metoprolol, acebutolol)[96] or drugs with intrinsic sympathomimetic activity (e.g., pindolol) may not interfere as much with the physiologic compensations for insulin-induced hypoglycemia.

EFFECTS ON BLOOD COAGULATION (TABLE 2-2)

Adrenergic stimuli may interact with the hemostatic processes at several points. Exercise or epinephrine administration causes a rapid rise in Factor VIII (antihemophilic globulin) levels, which can reach two to four times control level.[97] This increase can be totally blocked by propranolol or alprenolol but not by phenoxybenzamine or practolol.[98,99]

Propranolol has been shown to interfere with exercise-induced increments in fibrinolytic activity whereas practolol has no effect.[100]

In contrast to this potential detrimental effect on fibrinolysis some β-blockers have a potential beneficial effect on platelet activity. Excessive reactivity of blood platelets may contribute to arteriosclerotic vascular disease and its complications. The platelets of patients with thrombotic vascular disease show increased turnover rates and augmented responses to a variety of aggregating agents.[100-102] We have observed that the platelets of patients with angina pectoris have exaggerated aggregation responses which become normal during propranolol therapy.[102]

In in vitro experiments, propranolol (in concentrations similar to those safely achieved in vivo) abolished the second wave of human platelet aggregation induced by adenosine diphosphate (ADP) and epinephrine, and inhibited aggregation induced by collagen and thrombin.[103]

Propranolol blocked the release of ^{14}C-serotonin from platelets, inhibited platelet adhesion to collagen and interfered with clot retraction. Inhibition appeared unrelated to β-adrenergic blockade as (+)D-propranolol (which lacks β-blocking activity) was equipotent with (−)L-propranolol. Moreover, practolol, a β-blocking drug which is not membrane active (non-lipophilic), did not inhibit platelet function. These studies suggested that propranolol, like local anesthetics, decreases platelet responsiveness by a direct action on the platelet membrane. Modulation of platelet function by propranolol may occur at concentrations achieved with usual clinical doses of the drug.[103]

Oxprenolol[104] and pindolol, drugs with membrane activity, have also been shown to reduce platelet aggregability, though to a lesser degree than propranolol. If platelet hyperaggregability is contributory in atherosclerosis and its complications, then β-blockers, with effects on platelet membranes, may provide an extra protective effect in patients.

Recently, heightened platelet hyperaggregability has been described in patients with angina pectoris who had abrupt withdrawal of chronic therapy of propranolol. Whether or not platelet hyperresponsiveness contributes to the "rebound phenomenon" described with β-blocker withdrawal is provocative and warrants further investigation.[105, 106]

REFERENCES

1. Hansson L, Zweifler AJ, Julius S, Hunyor SN: Hemodynamic effects of acute and prolonged β-adrenergic blockade in essential hypertension. Acta Med Scand 196:27–34, 1974
2. Frolich ED: Hyperdynamic circulation and hypertension. Postgrad Med 52:64–73, 1972

3. Myers MG, Lewis PJ, Reid JL, Dollery CT: Brain concentration of propranolol in relation to hypotension effects in the rabbit with observations on brain propranolol levels in man. J Pharmacol Exp Ther 192:327-335, 1975
4. Reid JL, Lewis PJ, Myers MG, Dollery CT: Cardiovascular effects of intracerebroventricular d-, l- and dl-propranolol in the conscious rabbit. J Pharmacol Exp Ther 188:394-399, 1974
5. Offerhaus L, Van Zweiten PA: Comparative studies on central factors contributing to the hypotensive action of propranolol, alprenolol and their enantiomers. Cardiovasc Res 8:488-495, 1974
6. Laragh JH: Vasoconstriction-volume analysis for understanding and treating hypertension: the use of renin and aldosterone profiles. Am J Med 55:261-274, 1973
7. Winer N, Chekshi DS, Yoon MS, Freedman AD: Adrenergic receptor mediation of renin secretion. J Clin Endocrinol Metab 29:1168-1175, 1969
8. Michelakis AM, McAllister RG: The effect of chronic adrenergic receptor blockade on plasma renin activity in man. J Clin Endocrinol Metab 34:386-394, 1972
9. Tobert JA, Slater JDH, Fugelman F, et al.: The effect in man of (+) propranolol and racemic propranolol on renin secretion stimulated by orthostatic stress. Clin Sci 44:291-295, 1973
10. Weber MA, Stokes GS, Gain JM: Comparison of the effects of renin release of beta adrenergic antagonists with differing properties. J Clin Invest 54:1413-1419, 1974
11. Leonetti G, Mayer G, Morganti A, et al.: Hypotensive and renin suppressing activities of propranolol in hypertensive patients. Clin Sci Mol Med 48:491-499, 1975
12. Lydtin H, Schuchard J, Wober W, Dahlheim H, Thuran K: The effect of timolol on renin, angiotensin II, plasma catecholamines, and blood pressure in the human. In Magnani B (ed): Beta-Adrenergic Blocking Agents in the Management of Hypertension and Angina Pectoris. New York, Raven Press, 1974, p 81
13. Castenfors J, Johnson H, Oro L: Effects of alprenolol on blood pressure and plasma renin activity in hypertensive patients. Acta Med Scand 193:189-195, 1973
14. Kuramoto K, Kurihara H, Murata K, et al.: Haemodynamic effects and variations in plasma activity after oral administration of oxprenolol. J Intern Med Res 2:448-451, 1973
15. Stokes GS, Weber MS, Thornell IR: β-blockers and plasma renin activity in hypertension. Br Med J 1:60-62, 1974
16. Esler MD: Effect of practolol on blood pressure and renin release in man. Clin Pharmacol Ther 15:484-489, 1970
17. Waal-Manning HJ: Metabolic effects of β-adrenoceptor blockade. In Simpson FO (ed): Proceeding Queenstown Symposium. Drugs II:121-126, 1976
18. Waal-Manning HJ: Hypertension: which beta blocker? Drugs 12:412-441, 1976
19. Amery A, Billiet L, Fagard R: Beta receptors and renin release. N Engl J Med 290:284, 1974
20. Aberg H: Beta receptors and renin release. N Engl J Med 290:1025, 1974
21. Morgan TO, Roberts R, Carney SL, Louis WJ, Doyle AE: β-Adrenergic receptor blocking drugs, hypertension and plasma renin. Br J Clin Pharmacol 2:159-164, 1975
22. Krauss XH, Schalekamp MADH, Kolsters G, Zaal GA, Birkenhager WH: Effects of beta-adrenergic blockade on systemic and renal haemodynamic responses to hyper osmotic saline in hypertensive patients. Clin Sci 43:385-391, 1972

23. Prichard BNC: Propranolol as an antihypertensive agent. Am Heart J 79: 128-133, 1970

24. Imhof PR: Characterization of beta blockers as anti-hypertensive agents in the light of human pharmocology studies. In Schweizer W (ed): Beta-Blockers — Present Status and Future Prospects. Bern, Huber, 1974, pp 40-50

25. Waal HJ: Hypotensive action of propranolol. Clin Pharmacol Ther 7: 588-598, 1966

26. Rahn KH, Hawlina A, Kersting F, Planz G: Studies on the antihypertensive action of the optical isomers of propranolol in man. Naunyn Schmiedebergs Arch Pharmacol 286:319-323, 1974

27. Ahlquist RP: A study of the adrenotropic receptors. Am J Physiol 153:586-600, 1948

28. Sonnenblick EH, Ross J Jr, Braunwald E: Oxygen consumption of the heart. Newer concepts of its multifactorial determination. Am J Cardiol 22:328-336, 1968

29. Sonnenblick EH, Shelton CL: Myocardial energetics: Basic principles and clinical implications. New Engl J Med 285:668-675, 1971

30. Black JW, Stephenson JS: Pharmacology of a new adrenergic beta-receptor blocking compound (Nethalide). Lancet 2: 311-314, 1962

31. Robinson BF: Relation of heart rate and systolic blood pressure to the onset of pain in angina pectoris. Circulation 35:1073-1083, 1967

32. Wolfson S, Gorlin R: Cardiovascular pharmacology of propranolol in man. Circulation 40:501-511, 1969

33. Parratt JR, Grayson J: Myocardial vascular reactivity after β-adrenergic blockade. Lancet 1: 388-340, 1966

34. Becker LC, Fortuin NJ, Pitt B: Effects of ischemia and anti-anginal drugs on the distribution of radio-active microspheres in the canine left ventricle. Circ Res 28:263-269, 1971

35. Boakes AJ, Prichard BNC: The effects of AH 5158, pindolol, propranolol, and d- propranolol on acute exercise tolerance in angina pectoris. J Pharm Pharmacol 47:673-674, 1973

36. Barrett AM: A comparison of the effect of (±) propranolol and (+) propranolol in anesthetized dogs; β-receptor blocking and hemodynamic action. J Pharm Pharmacol 21: 241-247, 1969

37. Bjorntorp P: Treatment of angina pectoris with beta-adrenergic blockade, mode of action. Acta Med Scand 184: 259-262, 1968

38. Gianelly RS, Goldman RH, Treister B, Harrison DC: Propranolol in patients with angina pectoris. Ann Intern Med 67: 1216-1225, 1967

39. Prichard BNC: β-receptor antagonists in angina pectoris. Ann Clin Res 3: 344-352, 1971

40. Robinson BF: The mode of action of beta-antagonists in angina pectoris. Postgrad Med J 47(Suppl 2): 41-43, 1971

41. Morgan TO, Sabto J, Anavekar SM, Louis WJ, Doyle AE: A comparison of beta adrenergic blocking drugs in the treatment of hypertension. Postgrad Med J 50: 253-289, 1974

42. Connolly ME, Kersting F, Dollery CT: The clinical pharmacology of beta-adrenoceptor blocking drugs. Prog Cardiovasc Dis 19: 203-234, 1976

43. Prichard BNC, Aellig WH, Richardson GA: The action of intravenous oxprenolol, practolol, propranolol, and sotalol on acute exercise tolerance in angina pectoris: The

effect on heart rate and the electrocardiogram. Postgrad Med J 46: 77–85, 1970

44. Horn ME, Prichard BNC: Variable dose comparative trial of propranolol and sotalol in angina pectoris. Br Heart J 35: 555, 1973

45. Atkins JM, Blomqvist G, Cohen LS: Sotalol (MJ 1999) and propranolol in the treatment of angina pectoris. Clin Res 18:21, 1970

46. Toubes DB, Ferguson RH, Rice AJ: Beta adrenergic blockade vs. placebo in angina pectoris. Clin Res 18: 345, 1970

47. Brailovsky D: Timolol Maleate (MK-950), A new beta-blocking agent for the prophylactic management of angina pectoris. A multicentre, multinational, co-operative trial. In Magnani B (ed): Beta-adrenergic Blocking agents in the Management of Hypertension and Angina Pectoris New York: Raven Press, 1974, pp 117–137

48. Astrom H, Vallin H: Effect of a new beta adrenergic blocking agent, ici 66082 an exercise haemodynamics and airway resistance in angina pectoris. Br Heart J 36: 1194–1200, 1974

49. Roy P, Day L, Sowton E: Effect of new beta blocking agent, atenolol (Tenormin) on pain frequency, trinitrin consumption and exercise ability. Br Med J 3: 195–197, 1975

50. Hoffman BF, Singer DH: Appraisal of the effects of catecholamines on cardiac electrical activity. Ann NY Acad Sci 139: 914–939, 1967

51. Carmeliet E, Verdanok F: Interaction between ouabain and butridine, a beta-adrenergic blocking substance on the heart. Eur J Pharmacol, 1: 269–277, 1967

52. Han J: Mechanisms of ventricular arrhythmias associated with myocardial infarction. Am J Cardiol 24: 800–812, 1969

53. Singh BN, Jewitt DE: β-adrenoceptor blocking drugs in cardiac arrhythmias. In Avery G (ed.): Cardiovascular Drugs Vol 2. Baltimore, University Park Press, 1977, p 141–42

54. Levy JV, Richards V: Inotropic and chronotropic effects of a series of β-adrenergic blocking drugs: Some structure activity relationships. Proc Soc Exp Biol Med 122:373–379, 1966

55. Vaughan Williams EM, Papp J: The effect of oxprenolol on cardiac intracellular potentials in relation to its antiarrhythmia local anesthetic and other properties. Postgrad Med J 46: 22–32, 1970

56. Coltart DJ, Shand DG: Plasma propranolol levels in the quantitative assessment of β-adrenergic blockade in man. Br Med J 3: 731–734, 1970

57. Coltart DJ, Gibson DG, Shand DG: Plasma propranolol levels associated with suppression of ventricular ectopic betas. Br Med J 1: 490–495, 1971

58. Shand DG: Pharmacokinetic properties of beta-adrenergic blocking drugs. Drugs 7: 39–47, 1974

59. Jewitt DE, Singh BN: The role of beta-adrenergic blockade in myocardial infarction. Prog Cardiovasc Dis 16: 421–438, 1974

60. Gibson DG: Pharmacodynamic properties of beta-adrenergic receptor blocking drugs in man. Drugs 7: 8–38, 1974

61. Singh BN, Jewitt DE: Beta-adrenergic receptor blocking drugs in cardiac arrhythmias. Drugs 7: 426–461, 1974

62. Giudicelli JF, Lhoste F, Bossier JR: β-Adrenergic blockade and atrio-ventricular conduction impairment. Eur J Pharmacol 31: 216–225, 1975

63. Achong MR, Piafsky KM, Ogilvie RI: The effects of timolol (MK 950) and propranolol on peripheral vessels in man. Clin Pharmacol Ther 17: 228, 1975

64. Nies AS, McNeil JS, Schrier R: Mechanisms of increased sodium reabsorption during propranolol administration. Circulation 44: 596-604, 1976
65. Price HL, Cooperman LH, Warden JC: Control of the splanchnic circulation in man. Circ Res 21: 333-340, 1967
66. Meyer JS, Okamoto S, Shimazu K, et al.: Cerebral metabolic changes during treatment of subacute cerebral infarction by alpha and beta adrenergic blockade with phenoxybenzamine and propranolol. Strobe 5: 180-195, 1974
67. Packard RC: Uses of propranolol. N Engl J Med 293: 1205-1207, 1975
68. Oski FA, Miller LD, de Livoria A, et al.: Oxygen affinity in red cell changes induced in vivo by propranolol. Science 175: 1372-1373, 1972
69. Brain MC, Card RT, Kane J, et al.: Acute effects of varying doses of propranolol upon oxygen haemoglobin effects in man. Br J Clin Pharm 1: 67, 1974
70. Frishman W, Smithen C, Christodoulou J, et al.: Medical management of angina pectoris: Multifactorial action of propranolol. In Norman J, Cooley D (eds): Coronary Artery Medicine and Surgery. New York, Appleton, 1975, pp 285-295
71. Frishman W, Wilner G, Smithen C, Hayes J, Killip T: Effects of exercise and propranolol on hemoglobin oxygen affinity in patients with angina pectoris. Clin Res 24: 614, 1976
72. Frishman W, Davis R, Strom J, et al.: Clinical pharmacology of the new beta-adrenergic blocking drugs. Part 5. Pindolol (LB-46) therapy for supraventricular arrhythmia: A viable alternative to propranolol in patients with bronchospasm. Am Heart J 98: 393, 1979
73. Connolly CK, Batten JC: Comparison of the effect of alprenolol and propranolol on specific airway conductance in asthmatic patients. Br Med J 2: 515-615, 1970
74. Beumer HM, Hardonk HJ: Effects of beta adrenergic blocking drugs on ventilatory function in asthmatics. Eur J Clin Pharmacol. 5: 77-80, 1972
75. Bernecker C, Roetscher I: The beta blocking effect of practolol in asthmatics. Lancet 2: 662, 1970
76. Skinner C, Gaddo J, Palmer KNV: Comparison of effects of metoprolol and propranolol on asthmatic airway obstruction. Br Med J 1: 504, 1976
77. Skinner C, Palmer KNV, Kerridge DF: Comparison of the effects of acebutolol (Sectral) and practolol on airways obstruction in asthmatics. Br J Clin Pharmacol 2:417-422, 1972
78. Johnson G, Svedmyr M, Thirnger G: Effects of intravenous propranolol and metoprolol and their interaction with isoprenaline on pulmonary function, heart rate and blood pressure in asthmatics. Eur J Clin Pharmacol 8: 175-180, 1975
79. Kotler MN, Berinda L, Rubenstein AH: Hypoglycemia precipitated by propranolol. Lancet 2: 1389-1390, 1966
80. Deacon SP, Barnett D: Comparison of atenolol and propranolol during insulin-induced hypoglycemia. Br Med J 2: 272-273, 1976
81. Waal-Manning HJ: Metabolic effects of β-adrenoreceptor blockade. In Simpson FO (ed): Proceedings Queenstown Symposium. Drugs II:121-126, 1976
82. Lloyd-Mostyn RH, Oram S: Modification by propranolol of cardiovascular effects of induced hypoglycemia. Lancet 2: 1213-1215, 1975
83. Molnar GW, Read RC: Propranolol enhancement of hypoglycemic sweating. Clin Pharmacol Ther 15: 490-496, 1974

84. Porte D: Sympathetic regulation of insulin secretion. Its relation to diabetes mellitus. Arch Intern Med 123: 252–260, 1969

85. Antonis A, Clark MI, Hodge RL, Molony M, Pilkington TRE: Receptor mechanisms in the hyperglycemic response to adrenaline in man. Lancet 1: 1135–1137, 1967

86. Wray R, Sutcliffe SBJ: Propranolol-induced hypoglycaemia and myocardial infarction. Br Med J 2: 592, 1972

87. Podolsky S, Pattavina CG: Hyperosmolar non-ketotic diabetic coma: a complication of propranolol therapy. Metabolism 22: 685–693, 1973 ·

88. Blum I, Duren M, Laron Z, Atsmon A, Tiqua P: Prevention of hypoglycemic attacks by propranolol in a patient suffering from insomnia. Diabetes 24: 535–537, 1975

89. Loubatiere A, Mariani MM, Sorel G, Savi L: The action of β-adrenergic blocking drugs and stimulating agents on insulin secretion. Characteristics of the type of beta receptor. Diabetologica 7: 127–132, 1971

90. Allison SP, Chamberlain MJ, Miller JE, et al.: Effects of propranolol on blood sugar, insulin, and free fatty acids. Diabetologica 5: 339–342, 1969

91. Abramson EA, Arky RA, Woeber KA: Effects of propranolol on the hormonal and metabolic responses to insulin-induced hypoglycaemia. Lancet 2: 1386–1388, 1966

92. Harrison DC, Griffin JR: Metabolic and circulatory responses to selective adrenergic stimulation and blockade. Circulation 34: 218, 1974

93. Miller DW, Allen DO: Antilipolytic activity of 4- (2 hydroxy 3 isopropylaminopropoxy) acetanilide (practolol) Proceedings of the Society of Experimental Biology and Medicine. 136: 715, 1971

94. Mohs JM, Langley PE, Chase GR, Burns TW: In vivo observations on the rule of alpha and beta adrenergic receptor sites in human lipolysis. Clin Res 20: 57, 1972 (abs)

95. Sirtori CR, Azarnoff DL, Shoeman DW: Dissociation of the metabolic and cardiovascular effects of the beta-adrenergic blocker practolol. Pharmaceutical Research Communication 4: 123, 1972

96. Deacon SP, Karunanuyake A, Barnett D: Acebutolol, altenolol and propranolol and metabolic responses to acute hypoglycemia in man. Br Med J 2: 1255–1257, 1977

97. Cohn RJ, Epstein SE, Cohen LS, Dennis LH: Alterations of fibrinolysis and blood coagulation induced by exercise and the role of beta adrenergic blockade. Lancet 2: 1264–1266, 1968

98. Ingram GIC, Vaughan Jones R: The rise in clotting factor 8 induced in man by adrenaline. Effect of alpha and beta blockers. Physiol 187: 447–454, 1966

99. Gader AMA, da Costa J, Cash JD: The effect of propranolol, alprenolol, and practolol on the fibrinolytic and factor 8 responses to adrenaline and salbutamol in man. Thromb Res 2: 9–16, 1973

100. Steele PP, Weily HS, Davies H, Genton, E: Platelet function in coronary artery disease. Circulation 48: 1194–1200, 1973

101. Harker LA, Slichter S: Platelet and fibrinogen consumption in man. N Engl J Med 287: 999–1005, 1972

102. Frishman WH, Weksler B, Christodoulou JP, Smithen C, Killip T: Reversal of abnormal platelet aggregability and change in exercise tolerance in patients with angina pectoris following oral propranolol. Circulation 50: 887–896, 1974

103. Weksler BB, Gillick M, Pink J: Effect of propranolol on platelet function. Blood 49: 185–196, 1977

104. Rubegni M, Provedi D, Bellini PG, Bendinelli C, De Mauro G: Propranolol and platelet aggregation. Circulation 52: 964-965, 1975
105. Frishman WH, Christodoulou J, Weksler B, et al.: Abrupt propranolol withdrawal in angina pectoris. Effects on platelet aggregation and exercise tolerance. Am Heart J 95: 169-179, 1978
106. Frishman W, Weksler BB: Effects of beta-adrenoceptor blocking agents on platelet function in normal subjects and patients with angina pectoris. In International Symposium on Beta Adrenoceptor Blocking Drugs (1980). Amsterdam, Excerpta Medica, (in press)

CHAPTER THREE

Comparative Clinical Experience and New Therapeutic Applications

William H. Frishman and Ralph Silverman

BETA ADRENOCEPTOR blocking drugs have proved efficacious in the treatment of angina pectoris, hypertension, and cardiac arrhythmias. They have also shown clinical usefulness in the treatment of hypertrophic obstructive cardiomyopathies, hyperthyroidism, and pheochromocytoma. Clinical studies have suggested an even broader range of newer potential indications: migraine headache prophylaxis, anxiety states, schizophrenia, tremor, open-angle glaucoma, narcotic and alcohol withdrawal. There is also a growing debate whether β-adrenoceptor blocking drugs are useful in the therapy of acute myocardial infarction.

There have been many reports of clinical trials involving thousands of patients, most of which have dealt with propranolol, the drug in clinical use the longest. Clearly, no two studies were done under the same conditions or with the same experimental design, and the interpretation of their results is often difficult. Additionally, since so many physiologic variables are affected by the β-adrenergic system and hence, its blockade, the exact mode and nature of β-blocking effect in different clinical entities is nearly impossible to precisely define. However, an *overall* impression of the efficacy of these agents can be derived from results of clinical trials, and some of these results will be summarized for different pathophysiologic states. Some of the newer potential uses for β-adrenoceptor blocking drugs will also be discussed.

HYPERTENSION

There are several points to be noted in consideration of clinical trials with β-blockers in hypertension:

1. Patients may vary in individual dose requirements and rapidity of response. Hence, trials using small (or fixed) doses and short treatment periods may fail to show much effect.
2. In double-blind studies in which placebo follows active therapy, the duration of placebo therapy must be long enough to allow blood pressure to rise to pretreatment levels. If this is not done, then the therapeutic benefit of active drug will appear to be modest.
3. The best result of β-blockers in hypertension is achieved when they are used in combination with other drugs, especially diuretics.

Propranolol (Inderal). There is a vast experience with the use of propranolol in hypertensive patients, and hypertension is currenty a U.S. FDA approved indication for its use. Prichard and Gillam,[1] using propranolol in a large number of patients previously treated with other antihypertensive regimens, found that propranolol achieved the best control of supine blood pressure with the fewest side effects and the least postural hypotension. The average daily dose used was 319 mg with a maximum dose of 4,000 mg per day. Zacharias et al.[2] studied 109 patients, all of whom also received thiazide diuretics, and obtained good results in about 60 percent of his patients using an average dose of 290 to 320 mg per day (maximum 1000 mg per day). Only 20 percent of the patients required more than 600 mg per day. Other double blind trials in propranolol responders have shown a significant difference between drug and placebo.[3]

In a double-blind study of Jamaican blacks with hypertension, Humphreys and Delvin,[4] using lower doses of propranolol (maximum 360 mg per day) without diuretics, demonstrated far less satisfactory results. (This study raised the question of whether there is a decreased sensitivity of blacks to the effects of β-blockade than whites.)

In general, propranolol is now very widely used in hypertension. Its large usage in the United States prior to FDA approval for its use in hypertension testifies to the recognition of its efficacy by the medical community. Although generally effective, it frequently requires a high dosage, sometimes in the "gm" range.

Practolol (Eraldin). Practolol, the first cardiospecific β-blocker, has had widespread clinical use. It has fairly potent intrinsic sympathomimetic activity, but has no membrane-stabilizing activity. Many studies[5-10] have shown clinically significant reductions in blood pressure, and its cardioselectivity made it useful in patients felt to be at risk for developing asthma. The recognition of major toxic effects of practolol has led to its withdrawal, and the results of clinical trials will not be discussed further here.

Oxprenolol (Trasicor). Oxprenolol is a nonselective β-blocker, with partial agonist activity and less membrane effect than propranolol. Leishman et al.[5] studied the effect of oxprenolol in 14 patients. In a double-blind comparison between placebo and oxprenolol (320 mg per day, average), there was a significant reduction in supine and standing blood pressure with oxprenolol, without significant side effects. Tuckman,[11] in a study of 17 patients using an average daily dosage of 374 mg per day of oxprenolol (range 60 to 600 mg) also demonstrated reduction in systolic pressure without development of postural hypotension. Muiesan et al.[12] were able to demonstrate a dose-related antihypertensive effect for oxprenolol at much lower dosages (20 to 80 mg per day), when used in conjunction with hydrochlorthiazide and dihydralazine. Oxprenolol is equipotent, mg for mg, with propranolol.

Alprenolol (Aptin). Alprenolol is a nonselective β-blocker, with partial agonist activity (ISA) and some membrane activity. Tibblin and Åblad,[13] in a double-blind crossover comparison between alprenolol (up to 400 mg per day) and placebo in 11 patients, found significant reductions in supine and standing blood pressures with alprenolol, compared with placebo or control. Vedin et al.[14] found alprenolol, 400 to 800 mg per day, to be more effective than methyldopa, 750 to 1500 mg to day. Bengtsson[15] performed a double-blind comparision between alprenolol (150 to 300 μg tid) and propranolol (60 to 120 mg tid) in mild hypertensives. He found the two drugs to be equivalent, but there was less slowing of heart rate with alprenolol. In another double-blind crossover comparison of alprenolol (400 mg per day) and propranolol (60 mg per day), no significant difference could be demonstrated.[16] Chlorthalidone plus alprenolol (400 to 800 mg per day) and chlorthalidone plus methyldopa (750 to 1500 mg per day) produced similar beneficial effects in blood pressure reduction, but there were more severe side effects with methyldopa.[17] Overall alprenolol is very similar to oxprenolol.

Pindolol (Visken). Pindolol (prindolol) will be discussed in greater detail in a subsequent chapter. It has very little membrane activity and some possible peripheral vasodilator effect. Most prominent is its considerable intrinsic sympathomimetic activity, however, which may explain the paradoxical loss of blood pressure control seen in some patients in high dosages.

Pindolol is, mg for mg, the most potent of the β-blocking drugs. Several series have demonstrated good, often striking responses in blood pressure control, some at comparatively low doses.[18] In one trial of Waal-Manning and Simpson,[19] nearly all of 43 patients who were switched from other therapy to pindolol had improved blood pressure control, with an average dose of about 15 mg daily. Several other studies have also demonstrated clinically useful antihypertensive effects.[18] Pindolol has a longer duration of action than propranolol and can be given twice, or even once, daily with successful results.[20]

Sotalol (Betacardone, Sotacor). Sotalol is a noncardioselective β-blocker, without partial agonist activity (ISA) or membrane effect. It is effective in lowering blood pressure and is well-tolerated. Because its long half-life (9.5 hours), it need only be given twice daily. Sundquist et al.[8] found that on a weight basis, it is significantly less potent than propranolol, with an effect on blood pressure that is closely dose-related in doses of 200 to 600 mg per day.

Timolol (Blocadren). Timolol is a noncardioselective β-blocker with no intrinsic sympathomimetic or membrane-stabilizing activity (similar to sotalol). Dose for dose, it is about six times more potent than propranolol. It appears to be as effective a hypotensive agent as propranolol, and the recommended dose is 15 to 45 mg per day.[21,22]

Acebutolol (Sectral). Acebutolol has partial agonist activity and membrane-stabilizing effect. Although in animal studies it acts as a selective β-blocker, this has not been a general finding in man. It appears to be an effective antihypertensive agent, in doses up to 1000 mg per day.[23]

Atenolol (Tenormin). Atenolol is a cardioselective β-blocker with no intrinsic sympathomimetic activity or membrane-stabilizing activity. It has a comparatively long half-life: 6 hours. In a series of 43 patients using 100 mg of atenolol twice daily, Hansson et al.[24] were able to demonstrate excellent blood pressure responses with few side effects. They were able to confirm these initial results in a subsequent double blind comparison with placebo.[25] In a series of 37 patients treated with atenolol, Meekers et al.[26] found good results in almost all their patients, with little added benefit to be gained by doses higher than 300 mg per day.

Metoprolol (Betaloc, Lopresor). Metoprolol is a new cardioselective β-blocker without intrinsic sympathomimetic or membrane effect. In several studies,[27,28] it has been shown to be an effective, well-tolerated antihypertensive agent. It has recently been approved for use in hypertension by the U.S. FDA.

EFFICACY OF β-BLOCKERS IN HYPERTENSION

The β-blockers differ in terms of presence, or absence, of intrinsic sympathomimetic activity, membrane effect, cardioselectivity, and relative potencies and durations of action. It is unclear whether these differences have any practical relevance in the clinical treatment of hypertension: *all* β-blockers to date have antihypertensive effects. Three points, however, can be made: (1) drugs with intrinsic sympathomimetic activity (partial agonist activity) cause less bradycardia; (2) presence or absence of membrane-stabilizing effect seems to be irrelevant; (3) if a β-blocker has to be given to a potential asthmatic, it is best to use a selective β-blocker or one with ISA. (It must be cautioned, however, that as dosage increases, cardioselectivity diminishes.)

ANGINA PECTORIS

There is now no question about the effectiveness of β-adrenergic blockade in angina pectoris. Although the greatest experience has been with propranolol, therapeutic trials of other β-blocking agents have shown them also to be effective prophylactics. Although this chapter will not deal with the differences in clinical trial designs, it should be borne in mind that variations in design (run-in periods, fixed versus variable dosage schedules, duration of assessment period, acute versus chronic administration, etc.) may be responsible for differences in results obtained.

Propranolol (Inderal). There have been many trials of propranolol (membrane-stabilizing activity, no ISA, nonselective) with differing daily dosages that have demonstrated its effectiveness. The clinical efficacy of propranolol in angina is well known, and the results of clinical trials have been summarized by other authors.[29]

A dose-dependent reduction of anginal attacks with propranolol was well demonstrated in a study by Prichard and Gillam.[30] Sixteen patients were administered four different dose levels of propranolol and placebo, for a period of 2 weeks each, in a double-blind fashion. The average doses ranged from zero (placebo) to 417 mg per day. The initial study was repeated twice, thereby each patient receiving each treatment for 6 weeks. As dosage increased, there was a progressive decrease in the number of anginal attacks and in the amount of nitroglycerin used, giving a linear dose-response curve, whose slope, did not flatten even at the 417-mg dosage level (suggesting that maximum effect had not yet been obtained). Thus, if side effects do not intervene, patients can be expected to respond better on higher doses of propranolol than lower doses.

Oxprenolol (Trasicor). Membrane-stabilizing activity, intrinsic sympathomimetic activity, noncardioselectivity have been shown in trials. In a fixed dosage (80 mg tid) trial of oxprenolol, Sandler and Pistevos[31] failed to show a significant effect in 13 patients in frequency of angina attacks or in difference of exercise tolerance. Bianchi et al.[32] in 62 patients using a fixed dosage of 40 mg four times per day, demonstrated a decrease in frequency of angina and in nitroglycerin consumed. Both these studies used 2-week assessment periods and lacked proper run-in periods (the run-in period prior to the trial period proper provides times during which patients become familiar with the experimental protocol and during which drug dosage can be adjusted). Wilson et al.[33] performing a 2-week trial using a variable dose schedule (60 to 400 mg oxprenolol per day) that was preceded by a run-in period, demonstrated a significant benefit, with 17 of 18 patients having less angina with oxprenolol.

Alprenolol (Aptin). Trials demonstrated membrane-stabilizing activity, intrinsic sympathomimetic activity, and no cardioselectivity.

Wasserman et al.[34] studying 9 patients and using 4 weeks of treatment with 160 mg or 400 mg per day of alprenolol, failed to show a significant effect on anginal frequency of exercise tolerance. This trial did not have an adequate run-in period. Aubert et al.[35] using a fixed dose of 100 mg alprenolol 4 times per day, demonstrated a significant reduction in frequency of anginal attacks in 18 patients. Hickie,[36] using an 8-week run-in period in 50 patients in a multicenter trial, demonstrated a 33 percent reduction in number of attacks and nitroglycerin consumed with alprenolol compared with placebo. In a fixed multidose study, Sowton and Smithen[37] obtained an increase in exercise tolerance with doses of 100 mg, 200 mg, and 400 mg alprenolol twice daily. Although no dose-response relationship was demonstrated, this may reflect the design of the clinical trial (i.e., the administration of increasing drug dosages was not random) and is not conclusive.

Heatherington et al.[38] compared fixed doses of alprenolol (400 mg per day) and propranolol (160 mg per day) in 26 patients. Although there was increased exercise tolerance with both drugs, they both failed to provide a significant difference in frequency of anginal attacks and nitroglycerin consumption compared with placebo.

Pindolol (Visken). Trials demonstrated intrinsic sympathomimetic activity, no membrane-stabilizing effect, and no cardioselectivity.

Several double-blind studies have demonstrated that pindolol in a dose of 10 mg daily effected a greater decrease in anginal attacks and nitroglycerin consumation than placebo. Further discussion of pindolol, including results of our studies, is presented in Chapter 9.

Sotalol (Betacardone, Sotacor). Trials demonstrated no intrinsic sympathomimetic activity, no membrane-stabilizing activity, and no cardioselectivity.

In a fixed, multidose level (80, 160, 320, 640, 1280 mg sotalol per day) trial in 9 patients, Toubes et al.[39] demonstrated a significant decrease in frequency and severity of anginal attacks and a reduction in nitroglycerin consumption at all dose levels. In a variable oral dose trial comparing sotalol with propranolol, Horn and Prichard[40] found propranolol (average, 746 mg per day) to be more effective than sotalol (average 786 mg per day). This dose of sotalol was significantly better than low dose propranolol, however, (average, 93 mg per day).

Timolol (Blocarden) Trials showed no membrane-stabilizing activity, no ISA, and no cardioselectivity.

Brailovsky,[41] using an average dose of 30 mg timolol in a large multicenter trial in 307 patients, found a highly significant reduction in the frequency of anginal attacks compared with placebo.

Acebutolol (Sectral). Trials showed ISA and membrane-stabilizing effect; acts as a selective β-blocker in animals, but is questionable in man.

Khambatta[42] found acebutolol more effective than propranolol in a trial of 25 patients with angina pectoris. Since the dose of propranolol used in most of these patients was probably suboptimal (80 mg per day), however, it is difficult to draw firm conclusions from the study.

Practolol. Trials showed cardioselectivity with ISA.

Practolol was the first selective β-receptor antagonist developed. While used, it was found to be effective in angina pectoris. Because of increased recognition of toxic effects, practolol has been withdrawn from use and reports of clinical trials will not be discussed further here. In the past years, however, other cardioselective β-blockers have been developed.

Atenolol (Tenormin). Trials showed cardioselectivity and no ISA.

Aströmand Vallin[43] compared atenolol and propranolol, 5 mg intravenously, in 10 patients with severe angina. Both agents caused an equal reduction in exercise-induced tachycardia. Maximal work capacity was higher with atenolol; this may be related to its cardioselectivity, and, therefore, lack of interference with the peripheral vascular response to exercise. It was also observed that atenolol was associated with a slight increase in airway conductance, compared with the reduction produced by propranolol, which may also reflect cardioselectivity. Roy et al.[44] in a trial of 11 patients with severe angina, found that atenolol, in doses of 50, 100, and 200 mg twice daily, produced a significant reduction in anginal attacks and nitroglycerin consumption when compared with placebo. A dose-response relationship was also suggested by their results. There was some increase in exercise tolerance with atenolol that was not statistically significant.

Metoprolol (Betaloc, Lopressor). Trials showed cardioselectivity and no ISA.

Adolfsson et al.[45] in 17 patients given 40 mg metoprolol orally, demon-

strated a 42 percent increase in acute exercise tolerance. Other data also
seem to indicate that it is an effective antianginal agent.

It appears that β-blockers, when initiated at low dosage and when the
contraindications of asthma and congestive heart failure are observed, are a
safe and effective prophylaxis against angina pectoris. Although pain is
usually not totally relieved, the frequency of attacks is reduced and more
pain free exercise can be accomplished. Failure of chest pain to respond to
β-blocking drugs may be due to (1) poorly controlled heart failure with cardiac enlargement, (2) misdiagnosis of angina, or (3) inadequate dosage.
There is also some evidence, though not yet conclusive, that long-term β-
blockade improves prognosis, with some studies showing a decrease in mortality and rate of infarction.

ARRHYTHMIAS

β-Blocking drugs have become an important mode of treatment of various
cardiac arrhythmias. A discussion of their possible modes of action appears
in Chapter 2. Before discussing results of studies with some of these agents,
some general aspects of the individual arrhythmias in which β-blockade may
have a role, will be addressed. In general, β-blockers have been more effective in the treatment of supraventricular than of ventricular arrhythmias.

SUPRAVENTRICULAR ARRHYTHMIAS

These respond variably to β-blockade. They may often be as useful di-
agnostically as therapeutically: by slowing a very rapid heart rate, it sometimes will allow for the establishment of an accurate ECG diagnosis of an
otherwise puzzling arrhythmia.

SINUS TACHYCARDIA

This arrhythmia usually has an obvious cause (e.g., fever, hyperthyroidism, congestive heart failure, etc.), and therapy should address itself to
correction of the underlying condition. If the sinus tachycardia should require direct intervention, β-blockade is effective therapy.

SUPRAVENTRICULAR ECTOPICS

Again, treatment is seldom required and usually is addressed to the
underlying cause. These often herald the onset of atrial fibrillation, and
there is no evidence to show that β-blockade can prevent this development.

When due to digitalis toxicity, however, supraventricular ectopic beats generally respond well to β-blockade.

PAROXYSMAL SUPRAVENTRICULAR TACHYCARDIA (SVT)

These may be divided into two groups: (1) those related to abnormal conduction (e.g. reciprocating AV nodal tachycardia; the reentry tachycardias, as in Wolff-Parkinson-White syndrome, in which there is abnormal conduction through an AV nodal bypass pact), and (2) those caused by ectopic atrial activity, as in digitalis toxicity. Since β-blockade prolongs AV conduction, (A-H interval is increased in His bundle electrograms) and prolongs the refractory period of the reentrant pathways, it is no surprise that many cases of SVT respond to β-blockers. In acute episodes, vagal maneuvers after β-blockade may be effective in terminating the arrhythmia where they were unsuccessful before β-blockade. In addition, if sinus rhythm is still not restored, the use of β-blocking drugs still leaves the option of direct current countershock cardioversion, an option not safely available if digitalis is used initially.

ATRIAL FLUTTER

β-Blockade can be used to slow the heart (by increasing AV block) and may restore sinus rhythm. This is a situation in which β-blockade may be of diagnostic value: given intravenously, β-blockers slow the ventricular response and permit the differentiation of flutter waves, ectopic P-waves, or sinus mechanism.

ATRIAL FIBRILLATION

The major action of β-blockers here is the reduction in ventricular response by increasing the refractory period of the AV node. All β-blocking drugs have been effective in slowing ventricular rates in patients with atrial fibrillation. However, they are less effective than quinidine or DC cardioversion in the reversion of atrial fibrillation to sinus rhythm (although this can occur, especially when the atrial fibrillation is of recent onset). These drugs must be used cautiously when atrial fibrillation occurs in the setting of a severely diseased heart that is dependent on high levels of adrenergic tone to avoid failure. β-blockers may be particularly useful in controlling the ventricular rate in situations when this is difficult to achieve with maximum tolerated doses of digitalis. Examples are thyrotoxicosis and hypertrophic cardiomyopathy.

VENTRICULAR ARRHYTHMIAS

β-Blocking drugs can abolish or decrease the frequency of ventricular ectopic beats in various cardiac conditions. They are particularly useful if these arrhythmias are related to catecholamines (exercise, pheochromocytoma, halothane, anesthesia, exogenous administration of catecholamines) or digitalis. It has not been shown, however, that this reduces the incidence of sudden death from ventricular arrhythmia in patients at risk.

VENTRICULAR TACHYCARDIA AND FIBRILLATION

β-Blocking drugs should not be considered agents of choice in acute cases of ventricular tachycardia. Cardioversion or other antiarrhythmic drugs (lidocaine, quinidine, pronestyl, etc.) should be the initial agents of therapy. β-Blockers have, however, been shown to be of benefit in prophylaxis against recurrent ventricular tachycardia, particularly if sympathetic stimulation appears to be a precipitating cause. There have been many reported cases of prevention of exercise-induced ventricular tachycardia with β-blockers, in many of these cases there was a poor response to digitalis or quinidine.[47-50]

In ventricular fibrillation, although the immediate therapy is electrical defibrillation, intravenous administration of β-blocking drugs (in combination with lidocaine or pronestyl) may often be effective in preventing recurrences.[51,52]

As mentioned in Chapter 1, the effectiveness of β-blocking agents in arrhythmia seems to be related to cardiac β-adrenoreceptor blockade. Therefore, *all* β-blockers would be expected to be therapeutically effective in arrhythmias. If there is to be a preference for a given β-blocker in a specific situation, it would relate to its ease of administration, likelihood of side effects, and presence or absence of other associated properties (e.g., partial agonist activity, cardioselectivity).

Propranolol (Inderal). The efficacy of propranolol in the therapy of many cardiac arrhythmias is well established. Dosages of 80 to 100 mg 4 times daily, during chronic administration, are likely to produce plasma levels of 40 to 85 ng per ml or higher — a level that should be adequate for control of arrhythmias.[54,55] Occasionally, doses as low as 10 mg 4 times daily will provide good therapeutic results, therefore, it is reasonable clinical practice to start patients on a lower dosage regimen and gradually increase the dose until a satisfactory result is obtained.

Propranolol must be given cautiously by the intravenous route, especially when heart failure is present. One safe method is to give 0.5 to 0.75 mg every 2 minutes until the desired response is obtained or until a total dose of

0.1 mg per kg has been given. Blood pressure, electrocardiogram, and signs of congestive heart failure should be monitored and watched for, and atropine, isoproterenol and a temporary intravenous pacemaker wire should be available for use if bradycardia, AV block, or asystole should develop.

Alprenolol (Aptin). Alprenolol is similar to propranolol, in that it possesses comparable β-blocking and membrane stabilizing activity. It differs from propranolol in that alprenolol has significant intrinsic sympathomimetic activity (ISA, partial agonist activity). Because of its ISA, alprenolol does not depress resting heart rate or atrioventricular conduction as much as propranolol, and this may also provide less cardiac depressant activity, making it a potentially safer drug for use in impaired myocardial function.[56] An oral dose of 40 mg of propranolol has approximately equal β-blocking effect as 100 mg of alprenolol. Intravenously, the two drugs are approximately equipotent, mg for mg.

Many clinical studies have shown that the antiarrhythmic profile of alprenolol is similar to propranolol.[36,57-60] Fifty mg every 6 hours is a reasonable initial oral dose, which can be increased gradually to 100 mg or more every 6 hours until clinically adequate β-blockade is achieved. (A sustained release [200 mg tablet] preparation of alprenolol may be easier to administer and can be given every 12 hours). For acute therapy, alprenolol can be given intravenously at a rate of 1 mg per minute until the desired response is achieved or to a total of 20 mg.[60] Careful monitoring should be maintained, as with propranolol. In one series of 15 patients with acute myocardial infarction, 4 patients given alprenolol intravenously (2.5 to 5 mg) developed sudden circulatory collapse and clinical shock.[61]

Oxprenolol (Trasicor). Oxprenolol has about an equivalent β-blocking potency as propranolol, with less membrane-stabilizing effect and a significant partial agonist activity (intrinsic sympathomimetic activity). It has been used orally and intravenously in controlling cardiac arrhythmias[62,63] and can be used in a similar fashion as alprenolol. In acute therapy of arrhythmias, it may be given at a rate of one mg per minute up to a dose of 12 mg, using the previously described precautions. (Some authors have used up to 30 mg safely.[63]) Twenty mg every 6 hours appears to be a reasonable initial oral dose, which can be gradually increased as needed.

Pindolol (Visken). This β-blocker is being intensively evaluated, and details are discussed in Chapter 8. On a weight for weight basis, pindolol has been found to be from 4 to 40 times as potent a β-adrenoreceptor blocker as propranolol. It has very little membrane-stabilizing activity, but has significant intrinsic sympathomimetic activity and, therefore, will not depress resting heart rate as much as propranolol will.

Plasma levels effective in controlling arrhythmias (20 to 40 mg per ml) can be achieved by oral doses of 5 mg pindolol every 6 to 8 hours,[64] which provides antiarrhythmic activity similar to that of propranolol.[65] An intravenous total dose of 0.2 to 1.0 mg of pindolol is equivalent to 1 to 5 mg of IV propranolol, and provides an effective regimen for acute therapy. A dosage of 5 to 10 mg every 6 hours appears to be a suitable maintenance form of chronic oral therapy.

Practolol (Eraldin). Practolol is a cardioselective β-antagonist and was, therefore, felt to be a β-blocker of choice in patients with obstructive airways disease. (Cardioselectivity, however, is relative and decreases with larger doses which can, therefore, cause airway obstruction in some patients.[66]) It, like propranolol, has established value in the treatment of many cardiac arrhythmias.[67-69] Practolol has, however, been withdrawn from use because of serious toxic side effects, and will not be discussed further here.

Sotalol (Betacardone, Sotacor). Sotalol is a noncardioselective β-blocker without intrinsic sympathomimetic activity. It has no membrane-stabilizing activity, and has little myocardial depressant action. The antiarrhythmic spectrum of sotalol is similar to propranolol, practolol, or oxprenolol in doses up to 20 mg IV.[63,67,70-72] Sotalol may be a particularly useful agent in controlling arrhythmia related to elevated sympathetic activity, e.g., thyrotoxicosis, because it lacks intrinsic sympathomimetic properties.

Timolol (Blocadren). Timolol, which has no intrinsic sympathomimetic or membrane-stabilizing activity, is about 5 to 10 times as potent as propranolol in man. It seems to have antiarrhythmic effects comparable to those of propranolol.

Acebutolol (Sectral). Although it acts as a selective β-blocker in animals, this has been a variable finding in man. It possesses significant membrane stabilizing activity. Lewis et al.[73] have shown an antiarrhythmic spectrum for acebutolol similar to practolol, but acebutolol seems to have more myocardial depressant effect.

Atenolol (Tenormin). Atenolol is cardioselective, but differs from practolol in that it lacks intrinsic sympathomimetic activity. It has no membrane-stabilizing activity, and about half the β-blocking potency of propranolol. It has been shown to have antiarrhythmic properties comparable to propranolol.

Metoprolol (Betaloc, Lopressor). This is another cardioselective agent that is very similar to atenolol.

NEWER APPLICATIONS OF β-ADRENOCEPTOR AGENTS

HYPERTHYROIDISM

The role of the adrenergic nervous system in producing the features of thyrotoxicosis remains uncertain. Many of the features of the disease do resemble the effects of sympathetic stimulation and can be ameliorated although not totally abolished by spinal anesthesia, and ganglion blockade. In recent years, these observations have been extended to include the effect of β-adrenoceptor antagonists.[74] The results obtained have been conflicting. It is still not established whether the increased adrenergic activity is related either to increased levels of catecholamines or altered receptor sensitivity.[75-77] It is also possible, at least in the heart, that the changes might be attributed to a direct effect of thyroxine,[78] whose own nonspecific effectors (adenylate cyclase system) are separate from those of cardiac β-receptors.[79]

Despite the failure to elucidate precisely the relationship between hyperthyroidism and catecholamines, the apparent clinical connection has resulted in attempts to induce sympathetic blockade as part of the management of the disease for many years. Sympatholytic drugs, quanethidine, and methyldopa were first used and subsequently, pronethalol, the first β-adrenoceptor blocking drug, was given to patients with spontaneous hyperthyroidism, all without much apparent useful effect.[80] Propranolol was shown, however, to reduce resting heart rate signficantly in hyperthyroid patients and subsequent β-blocking drugs, in particular propranolol, have been extensively investigated in this disease.[81]

The exact mechanism of β-blockers in hyperthyroidism is not fully defined. It is not fully known whether the effects of β-blockers are mediated through an adrenergic blockade mechanism, or as has recently been suggested, by blocking the peripheral conversion of T4 to T3.[82]

Particular benefit has been obtained with β-blocking in the management of thyrotoxic crises (thryoid storm).[83] β-Blockade produces a rapid reduction in fever, tachycardia, and central effects, such as restlessness and disorientation. Most of the experience to date with β-blockers in "thyroid storm" has been reported with propranolol.[84] β-Blockers have also been used as a preoperative medication in thyrotoxic patients undergoing partial thyroidectomy.[85]

As part of the routine medical management, β-blocking drugs are of less certain value. All are capable of reducing heart rate, although pronethalol, oxprenolol, alprenolol, practolol, and pindolol (all of which possess intrinsic sympathomimetic activity) are less effective than those agents without this property (such as propranolol and sotalol). Other manifestations of the disease such as tremor, hyperreflexia, agitation, hemodynamic changes, hyperkinesia, and those eye signs attributable to sympathetically innervated smooth muscle, all may be reduced by propranolol, practolol, sotalol, and pindolol.[86-90]

β-Blockade in thyrotoxic patients has no effect on either thyroid hormone secretion, the peripheral disposal of thyroxine, or the thyrotropic and prolactin responses to thyrotropin-releasing hormone.[91] Patients fail to gain weight satisfactorily, although an improved nitrogen balance and evidence of increased metabolism persists.[78,87,92,93] β-Blockers cannot be considered as long-term substitutes for specific antithyroid therapy.

In establishing the role for β-blockers in hyperthyroidism, drugs with intrinsic sympathomimetic activity are effective in reducing the peripheral manifestations of hyperthyroidism, but they are less effective than drugs without intrinsic sympathomimetic activity, particularly with respect to control of tachycardia. Further experience has not confirmed the early contention that drugs with intrinsic sympathomimetic activity might be responsible for precipating arrhythmias in hyperthyroid patients and might, therefore, be dangerous.[94]

HYPERTROPHIC CARDIOMYOPATHY

β-Adrenoceptor blocking drugs have proved to be efficacious in the therapy of patients with hypertrophic cardiomyopathy or idiopathic hypertrophic subaortic stenosis (IHSS).[95-96] These drugs are useful in controlling the symptoms: dyspnea, angina, and syncope.[97] They also have been shown objectively to lessen the intraventricular pressure gradient both at rest and with exercise.

The outflow pressure gradient is not the only abnormality in hypertrophic cardiomyopathy; more important is the loss of ventricular compliance which impedes left ventricular function. It has been shown by invasive and noninvasive methods that both propranolol and practolol improve left ventricular function.[98] Both drugs produce favorable changes in ventricular compliance and reduction of angina and palpitations.

The long-term hemodynamic effects of β-blockers have not been established but since these agents have such a beneficial effect on impaired ventricular compliance, they may frequently influence the natural history of the disease.

There has been limited experience, except for anecdotal situations, with the other β-blockers (other than practolol) in therapy of hypertrophic cardiomyopathy. One might suspect, however, that an agent with intrinsic sympathomimetic activity might be less efficacious than a β-blocker without this property. This was suggested by a lesser improvement with practolol as compared to propranolol in a study of patients with hypertrophic cardiomyopathy.[98]

MYOCARDIAL INFARCTION

There is some evidence that administration of β-adrenoceptor blocking agents shortly after the onset of acute myocardial infarction might decrease the amount of ischemic injury in selected individuals. The drugs' precise roles in the treatment and prophylaxis of acute myocardial infarction and its recurrence, however, is controversial and requires additional research and study. This subject will be discussed in greater detail in Chapter 7.

NEWER THERAPEUTIC INDICATIONS FOR β-BLOCKERS

Migraine Prophylaxis. Several studies have demonstrated the prophylaxis efficacy of propranolol for migraine headache.[99,100] About a third of the patients in these studies showed dramatic improvement in frequency and severity of attacks, along with a significantly reduced need for ergotamine and analgesic medication. Another third of the patients showed moderate improvement and the remainder showed no response to propranolol therapy.

Inhibition of peripheral vasodilation is the likely reason for the beneficial effect of propranolol in migraine. Pindolol and alprenolol, perhaps because of their partial agonist activity, have shown little or no effect in migraine.[101]

Tremor. There is some evidence that heightened adrenergic activity may play a role in some varieties of tremor.[102,103] Propranolol is reportedly useful in the treatment of action tremors, including essential, familial, and senile tremors, and familial essential myoclonus.[104–106] Most of the patients with benign action tremors noted clinical improvement with 60 to 240 mg of oral propranolol daily. A few patients showed virtually complete resolution of the tremor, while the majority of the patients reported mild improvement. The best responses were obtained in younger patients who had shorter histories of tremor. In one long-term study, the drug did not prevent the gradual progression of essential tremor, but clinical improvement was still apparent after 2 to 4 years of continuous propranolol treatment.

There are as yet no good clinical studies using the newer β-blocking drugs for treatment of tremor. Whether or not nonselective β-blockers will prove more efficacious than those with cardioselectivity has yet to be determined.

Anxiety. Granville-Grossman[107] first suggested that β-blocking drugs might be of value in treating anxiety. Since that time several studies have appeared and most of them have been reviewed by Whitlock and Price.[108] Overall, the studies are rather inconclusive even when the investigators utilize a satisfactory double-blind protocol. It was found that patients derived benefit from propranolol only if they presented initially with dominant somatic complaints, (palpitations, shakiness, tremor) as opposed to psychic symptoms. β-Blockers effect the physiologic consequences of anxiety probably by blockage of a peripheral feedback loop of sympathetically mediated responses.[109]

Noncardioselective β-blockers (propranolol, alprenolol), might be more useful in anxiety states than drugs with cardioselectivity (which do not block peripheral receptors) or intrinsic sympathomimetic activity (which activate peripheral receptors). This has not yet been tested in clinical trials, however.

Schizophrenia. The use of β-adrenoceptor blocking drugs in this area is highly controversial.[108,110] Several studies have appeared that describe the use of propranolol (up to 5800 mg per day) in schizophrenic patients.[111,112]

In general, favorable results have been claimed in patients with acute psychotic states, while chronically affected patients do not seem to respond. The beneficial response to β-blockade becomes apparent sometimes within hours.[110]

Despite the initial excitement generated by the apparent usefulness of β-blockers in acute psychosis, none of the clinical trials were based on double-blind design. The possibility of spontaneous clinical remission and the concomitant use of other antipsychotic drugs were not taken into consideration.[113] The possible mechanism for a β-blocker response in patients with acute schizophrenia has also not yet been elucidated. If it relates to a central nervous system effect, those drugs which rapidly cross the blood–brain barrier (alprenolol, propranolol) might prove more efficacious than β-adrenoceptor blocking agents which do not demonstate this property.

Narcotic and Alcohol Withdrawal. Anecdotal reports suggest that propranolol reduces heroin-induced euphoria, ameliorates narcotic abstinence syndromes, and may be useful in treating narcotic addiction.[114,115] However, no adequate clinical trials have been conducted with propranolol or the other new β-adrenoceptor blocking agents in treating narcotic addiction, and the effectiveness of these drugs in this condition is questionable.

Propranolol has been successfully used to manage patients undergoing acute alcohol withdrawal.[116] The drugs effect on alcohol withdrawal symptoms is thought to be due to blockade of central nervous system β-adrenoceptors with a subsequent decrease in sympathetic outflow. Patients with mild to moderate symptoms of alcohol withdrawal responded to 40 to 160 mg of oral propranolol daily over 6 days of therapy. Agitation and tremors lessened, none of the patients developed delirium tremens or withdrawal seizures, and all tolerated the drug well. At the time of this writing there has been no published experience with the newer β-adrenoceptor-blocking drugs for this indication.

Open-Angle Glaucoma. Timolol maleate (Timoptic), a β-adrenergic receptor blocking agent (noncardioselective) for ophthalmic administration, was recently approved by the U.S. FDA for treatment of chronic open-angle glaucoma. It is also approved for aphakic glaucoma and for some patients with secondary glaucoma.

As early as 1967, propranolol was shown to decrease intraocular pressure.[117] However, its mild anesthetic properties made investigators reluctant to use it as topical medication for glaucoma. Timolol does not have this local anesthetic activity, and has a beta blocking potency five to ten times that of propranolol on a mg to mg basis.

Zimmerman and Kaufman[118] studied patients with chronic open-angle glaucoma treated with 0.5 percent and 1.5 percent timolol. The patients exhibited decreased intraocular pressure in both treated and untreated eyes for the entire 7 hours that the pressures were measured.

Slowing of the heart rate can occur, presumably due to systemic absorption.[117] It is recommended that timolol be prescribed with caution for patients with known contraindications to systemic use of β-adrenergic receptor blocking agents such as asthma, heart block, or heart failure.

REFERENCES

1. Prichard BNC, Gillam PMS: Treatment of hypertension with propranolol. Br Med J 1:7-16, 1969
2. Zacharias FJ, Cowen KJ, Prestt J, Vickers J, Wall BG: Propranolol in hypertension: a study of long-term therapy, 1964-1970. Am Heart J 83:755-761, 1972
3. Zacharias FJ, Cowen KJ: Controlled trial of propranolol in hypertension. Br Med J 1: 471-474, 1970
4. Humphreys GS, Delvin DG: Ineffectiveness of propranolol in hypertensive Jamaicans. Br Med J 2:601-603, 1968
5. Leishman AWD, Thirlettle JL, Allen BR, Dixon RA: Controlled trial of oxprenolol and practolol in hypertension. Br Med J 4:342-344, 1970
6. Prichard BNC, Boakes AJ, Day G: Practolol in the treatment of hypertension. Postgrad Med J 47 (Suppl):84-92, 1971
7. Esler MD, Nestel PJ: Evaluation of practolol in hypertension. Effects on sympathetic nervous system and renin responsiveness. Br Heart J 35:469-474, 1973
8. Sundquist H, Anttila M, Arstila M: Antihypertensive effects of practolol and sotalol. Clin Pharmacol Ther 16:465-472, 1974
9. Waal-Manning, HJ: Comparative studies on the hypotensive effects of beta-

adrenergic receptor blockade. In Simpson, FO: Symposium on Beta-adrenergic Receptor Blocking Drugs. Auckland, CIBA, 1970 p 64

10. Galloway DB, Beattie AG, Petrie JC: Practolol and bendrofluazide in treatment of hypertension. Br Heart J 36:867–871, 1974

11. Conolly ME, Kersting F, Dollery CT: The clinical pharmacology of beta-adrenoreceptor-blocking-drugs. Prog Cardiovasc Dis 19:203–234, 1976

12. Muiesan G, Motolese M, Colombi A: Hypotensive effect of oxprenolol in mild hypertension: a cooperative controlled study. Clin Sci Mole Med 45:163s–166s, 1973

13. Tibblin G, Ablad B: Antihypertensive therapy with alprenolol, a b-adrenergic receptor antagonist. Acta Med Scand 186:451–457, 1969

14. Vedin JS, Wilhelmsson CE, Werkö L: Comparative study of alprenolol and methyldopa in previously untreated essential hypertension. Br Heart J 35:1285–1292, 1973

15. Bengtsson C: Comparison between alprenolol as antihypertensive agents. A double-blind cross-over study. Acta Med Scand 192:415–417, 1972

16. Somer T, Luomanmaki K, Frick MH: Alprenolol and propranolol in the treatment of hypertension: A comparative study. Acta Med Scand (Suppl 554):33–37, 1974

17. Tuomilehto J, Puska P, Mustaniemi H: A comparative study of alprenolol and alpha methyldopa respectively in combination with chlorthalidone in hypertension. Acta Med Scan (Suppl 554):47–54, 1974

18. Simpson FO: b-adrenoreceptor blocking drugs in hypertension. In Avery (ed), b-adrenoreceptor Drugs. Baltimore, University Park Press, 1978, pp 62–63

19. Waal-Manning HJ, Simpson FO: Pindolol: a comparison with other antihypertensive drugs and a double blind placebo trial. NZ J Med 80:151–157, 1974

20. Waal-Manning HJ, Wood AJ: Pindolol in hypertension twice daily versus thrice daily dosage. Med J Aust 2:274–275, 1975

21. Franciosa JA, Freis ED, Conway J: Antihypertensive and hemodynamic properties of the new beta-adrenergic blocking agent timolol. Circulation 48:118–124, 1973

22. Lohmöller G, Frolich ED: A comparison of timolol and propranolol in essential hypertension. Am Heart J 89:437–442, 1974

23. Letal B, Fillashe LP, Wolff LM: The treatment of essential hypertension with acebutolol. Clin Trials J 3:92–95, 1974

24. Hansson L, Henningsen NC, Karlberg B, et al.: Hypertensive action of ICI 66.082, A new beta-adrenergic blocking agent. Int J Clin Pharmacol Ther Toxicol 10:206–211, 1974

25. Hansson L, Aberg H, Karlberg BE, Westerlund A: Controlled study of atenolol in treatment of hypertension. Br Med J 2:367–370, 1975

26. Meekers J, Missotten A, Fagard R, et al.: Predictive value of various parameters for the antihypertensive effect of the beta blocker ICI 66.082. Arch Intern De Pharmacodynamie et de Therapie 213:294–306, 1975

27. Bengtsson C, Johnsson G, Regardh CG: Plasma levels and effects of metoprolol on blood pressure and heart rate in hypertensive patients after an acute dose and between two doses during long-term treatment. Clin Pharmacol Ther 17:400–408, 1975

28. Waal-Manning HJ: Clinical trial of metoprolol (H93/26) in hypertension. NZ J Med 82:138, 1975

29. Prichard BNC: β-adrenoceptor blocking drugs in angina pectoris. In Avery (ed): β-Adrenoceptor Blocking Drugs. Sydney, Australia, ADIS, 1978, pp 85-118

30. Prichard BNC, Gillam DMS: An assessment of propranolol in angina pectoris. A clinical dose response curve and the effect on the electrocardiogram at rest and on exercise. Br Heart J 33:473-480, 1971

31. Sandler G, Pistevos A: Clinical evaluation of oxprenolol in angina pectoris. Br Heart J 34:847-850, 1972

32. Bianchi C, Lucchello PE, Starcich R: Beta-blockade and angina pectoris. A controlled multicentre clinical trial. Pharmacologica Clinica 1:161-167, 1969

33. Wilson DF, Watson OF, Peel JS, Turner AS: Trasicor in angina pectoris: a double-blind trial. Br Med J 2: 155-157 1969

34. Wasserman AJ, Proctor JD, Allen FJ, Kemp VE: Human cardiovascular effects of alprenolol, a beta-adrenergic blocker: Haemodynamic, anti-arrhythmic, and antianginal. J Clin Pharmocol 10:37-49, 1970

35. Aubert A, Nyberg G, Slaastad R, Tjeldflaat L: Prophylactic treatment of angina pectoris. A double-blind cross-over comparison of alprenolol and pentanitrol. Br Med J 1:203-206, 1970

36. Hickie JB: Alprenolol (Aptin) in angina pectoris. A double-blind multicentre trial. Med J Aust 2:268-272, 1970

37. Sowton E, Smithen C: Double-blind three-dose trial of oral alprenolol in angina pectoris. Br Heart J 33:601-606 1971

38. Heatherington DJ, Comerford MB, Nyberg G, Besterman EMM: Comparison of two adrenergic beta-blocking agents, alprenolol and propranolol, in the treatment of angina pectoris. Br Heart J 35:320-333, 1973

39. Toubes DB, Ferguson RK, Rice AJ, et al.: β-adrenergic blockade vs. placebo in angina pectoris. Clin Res 18:345, 1970

40. Horn E, Prichard BNC: A variable dose comparative trial of propranolol and sotalol in angina pectoris. Br Heart J 35:555, 1973

41. Brailovsky D: Timolol maleate (ML-950). A new beta-blocking agent for the prophylactic management of angina pectoris. A multicentre, multinational, co-operative trial. In Magnani B (ed): Beta-adrenergic Blocking Agents in the Management of Hypertension and Angina Pectoris. New York, Raven Press, 1974, pp 117-137

42. Khambatta RB: Comparison of a new β-receptor blocking agent acebutolol (Sectral) and propranolol. Clin Trials 11 (Suppl 3):59-67, 1974

43. Astrom H, Vallin H: Effects of a new beta adrenergic blocking agent, ICI 66082, on exercise haemodynamics and airway resistance in angina pectoris. Br Heart J 36: 1194-1200, 1974

44. Roy P, Day L, Sowton E: Effect of new β-adrenergic blocking agent, atenolol (Tenormin), on pain frequency, trinitrin consumption and exercise ability. Br Med J 3:195-197, 1975

45. Adolfsson L, Areskog NH, Furberg C, Johnsson G: Effects of single doses of alprenolol and two cardioselective β-blockers (H 87/07 and H 93/26) on exercise induced angina pectoris. Eur J Clin Pharmacol 7:111-118, 1974

46. Frishman W, Silverman R: Clinical pharmacology of the new beta adrenergic blocking drugs (part 2): Physiologic and metabolic effects. Am Heart J 97: 797, 1979

47. Taylor RR, Halliday EJ: Beta-adrenergic blockade in the treatment of exercise-induced paroxysmal ventricular tachycardia. Circulation 32:778-782, 1965

48. Sloman G, Stannard M: Beta-adrenergic blockade and cardiac arrhythmias. Br Med J 4:508-512, 1967
49. Gettes LS, Surawicz B: Long-term prevention of paroxysmal arrhythmias with propranolol therapy. Am J Med Sci 254:257-265, 1967
50. Wennevold A, Sandoe E: Propranolol (Inderal) in the long-term prophylaxis of ventricular arrhythmias. Acta Med Scand 183:87-93, 1968
51. Ikram H: Propranolol in persistent ventricular fibrillation complicating acute myocardial infarction. Am Heart J 75:795-796, 1968
52. Sloman G, Robinson JS, McLean K: Propranolol (Inderal) in persistent ventricular fibrillation. Br Med J 1:895-899, 1965
53. Frishman W: Clinical pharmacology of the new beta-adrenergic blocking drugs (part 1): Pharmacodynamic and pharmacokinetic properties. Am Heart J 97:663, 1979.
54. Coltart DJ, Shand DG: Plasma propranolol levels in the quantitative assessment of beta-adrenergic blockade in man. Br Med J 3:731-735, 1970
55. Coltart DJ, Gibson DG, Shand DG: Plasma propranolol levels associated with suppression of ventricular ectopic beats. Br Med J 1:490-495, 1971
56. Ablad B, Brogard M, Ek L: Pharmacological properties of H56/28 — a beta-adrenergic receptor antagonist. Acta Pharmacol Toxicol 25 (Suppl 2):9-40, 1967
57. Linko E, Siitonen L, Ruosteenoja R: A new beta-adrenergic receptor blocking agent. H56/28, in the treatment of cardiac arrhythmias. Acta Med Scand 181:547-552,1967
58. Anthony JR, Jick H, Spodick DH: Control of persistent ventricular ectopic beats by alprenolol, a new beta-blocking agent. Am Heart J 77:598-602, 1969
59. Kerber RE, Goldman RH, Gianelly RE, Harrison DC: Treatment of atrial arrhythmias with alprenolol, JAMA 214:1849-1854, 1970
60. Lemberg L, Arcebal AG, Castellanos A, Slavin D: Use of alprenolol in acute cardiac arrhythmias. Am Heart J 30:77-81, 1972
61. Kreus KE, Salokannel SJ, Isomaki H, Waris EK: Alprenolol in the treatment of arrhythmias in acute coronary patients. Acts Med Scand 188:375-378, 1970
62. Fuccella LM, Imhoff P: Experience with a new beta-receptor blocking agent (Transicor) in the management of cardiac arrhythmias. Pharmacol Clin 1:123-130, 1969
63. Sandler G, Pistevos AC: Use of oxprenolol in cardiac arrhythmias associated with acute myocardial infarction. Br Med J 1:254-257, 1971
64. Storstein L: LB-46, a new beta-adrenergic receptor blocking agent in cardiac arrhythmias. Acta Med Scand 191:423-428, 1972
65. Aronow WS, Uyeyama RR: Treatment of arrhythmias with pindolol. Clin Pharmacol Ther 13:15-22, 1972
66. Waal-Manning HJ, Simpson FO: Practolol treatment in asthmatics. Lancet 2:1264-1265, 1971
67. Jewitt DE, Mercer CJ, Hubner PJ, Shillingford JP: Comparison of drugs used in management of arrhythmias developing after acute myocardial infarction. Br Heart J 31:794-802, 1969
68. Allen JD, Pantridge JF, Shanls RG: Practolol in the treatment of ventricular dysrhythmias in acute myocardial infarction. Postgrad Med J 47 (Suppl Jan):29-34, 1971
69. Jewitt DE, Croxson R: Practolol in the management of cardiac dysrhythmias following myocardial infarction and cardiac surgery. Postgrad Med J 47 (Suppl. January): 25-30, 1971
70. Theilen EO, Wilson WR: Beta-adrenergic receptor blocking drugs in the treatment

of cardiac arrhythmias. Med Clin North Am 52:1017-1029, 1968

71. Fogelman F, Lightman SL, Sillet RW, McNicol MW: The treatment of cardiac arrhythmias with sotalol. Eur J Clin Pharmacol 5:72-76, 1972

72. Prakash P, Allen AN, Kondo F, et al.: Clinical evaluation of the anti-arrhythmic effects of sotalol (MJ1999). Am J Cardiol 26:654, 1970

73. Lewis BS, Mitha AS, Gotsman MS: Acebutolol in cardiac arrhythmias. South Afr Med J 20:821-824, 1974

74. Dollery CT, Paterson JW, Conolly MR: Clinical phamacology of beta receptor blocking drugs. Clin Pharmacol Ther 10:765-799, 1969

75. Levey GS: Catecholamine hypersensitivity, thyroid hormone and the heart — a reevaluation. Am J Med 50:413-420, 1971

76. Brewster WR, Isaacs JP, Osgood PF, King TL-RN: The hemodynamic and metabolic interrelationships in the activity of epinephrine, norepinephrine and the thyroid hormones. Circulation 13:1-20, 1956

77. Ramsay I: Adrenergic beta blockade in hyperthyroidism. Br J Clin Pharmacol 2:385-388, 1975

78. Grossman W, Robin NI, Johnson LW, Brooks HL, Selenkow HA: The enhanced myocardial contractility of the thyrotoxicosis-role of the beta adrenergic receptor. Ann Intern Med 74:869-874, 1971

79. Levey GS, Epstein SE: Myocardial adenyl cyclase: Activation by thyroid hormones and evidence for two adenyl cyclase systems. J Clin Invest 48:1663-1669, 1969

80. Wilson WR, Theilin EO, Fletcher FW: Pharmacodynamic effects of beta-adrenergic receptor blockade in patients with hyperthyroidism. J Clin Invest 41:1697-1703, 1967

81. Rowlands DJ, Howitt G, Markham P: Propranolol (Inderal) in disturbances of cardiac rhythm. Br Med J 2:891-894, 1965

82. Wiersinga WM, Touber JL: The influence of b-adrenoceptor blocking drugs on plasma thyroxine and triiodothyronine. J Clin Endocrinol Metab 45:293-298, 1977

83. Das G, Krieger M. Treatment of thyrotoxic storm with intravenous adminstration of propranolol. Ann Intern Med 70:985-988, 1969

84. Lee TC, Coffey RJ, Mackin J, et al.: The use of propranolol in the surgical treatment of thyrotoxic patients. Ann Surg 177:643-647, 1973

85. Pimstone BL: Beta adrenergic blockade in thyrotoxicosis. S Afr Med J 43 (Suppl Dec 6): 27-29, 1969

86. Turner P: Alprenolol and propranolol in hyperthyroid tachycardia. Br J Pharmacol 40:146, 1970

87. Schelling JL, Scazziga B, Dufour RJ, Milinkovic N, Wever AA: Effect of pindolol, a beta receptor antagonist, in hyperthyroidism. Clin Pharmacol Ther 14:158-164, 1973

88. Shanks RG, Hadden DR, Lowe DC, McDevitt DG: Controlled trial of propranolol in thyrotoxicosis. Lancet 1:993-994, 1969

89. Nelson JK, McDevitt DG: Comparative trial of propranolol and practolol in hyperthyroidism. Br J Clin Pharmacol 2:411-416, 1975

90. Grossman W, Robin NI, Johnson LW, Brooks H, Selenkow A: The effect of beta blockade on the peripheral manifestation of thyrotoxicosis. Ann Intern Med 74:875-879, 1971

91. Wartofsky L, Dimond RC, Noel GL, Frantz AG, Earll JM: Failure of propranolol to alter thyroid iodine release, thyroxine turnover, or the TSH and PRL responses to thyrotropin-releasing hormone in patients with thyrotoxicosis. J Clin Endocrinol

Metab 41:485–490, 1975

92. Pimstone B, Joffe B: The use and abuse of beta adrenergic blockade in the surgery of hyperthyroidism. S Afr Med J 44:1059–1061, 1970

93. Georges LP, Santangelo RP, Mackin JF, Canary JJ: Metabolic effects of propranolol in thyrotoxicosis. 1: Nitrogen, calcium and hydroxyproline. Metabolism 24:11–23, 1975

94. Turner P, Hill RC: A comparison of three beta-adrenergic receptor blocking drugs in thyrotoxic tachycardia. J Clin Pharmacol 8:268–271, 1968

95. Goodwin JF: The congestive and hypertrophic cardiomyopathies — a decade of study. Lancet 1:731–739, 1970

96. Matlof HJ, Harrison DC: Acute haemodynamic effects of practolol in patients with idiopathic hypertrophic subaortic stenosis. Br Heart J 35:152–158, 1973

97. Cherian G, Brockington IM, Shah PM, Oakley EM, Goodwin JF: Beta-adrenergic blockade in patients with hypertrophic obstructive cardiomyopathy. Am Heart J 73: 140–141, 1967

98. Hubner PJB, Ziady GM, Lane GK, et al.: Double-blind trial of propranolol and practolol in hypertrophic cardiomyopathy. Br Heart J 35:1116–1123, 1973

99. Weber RB, Reinmuth O: The treatment of migraine with propranolol. Neurology 22:366–369, 1972

100. Stensrod P, Sjaastad O: Short-term clinical trial of propranolol in racemic form (Inderal); d-propranolol and placebo in migraine. Acta Neurol Scand 53:229–232, 1976

101. Packard RC: Uses of propranolol. N Engl J Med 293:1205, 1975

102. Marsden CD, Foley TH, Owen DAL, McAllister RG: Peripheral beta-adrenergic receptors concerned with tremor. Clin Sci 33:53–65, 1967

103. Young RR, Growdon JH, Shahani BT: Beta adrenergic mechanisms in action tremor. N Engl J Med 293:950–953, 1975

104. Murray TJ: Long-term therapy of essential tremor with propranolol. Can Med Assoc J 115:892–894, 1976

105. Winkler GF, Young RR: Efficacy of chronic propranolol therapy in action tremors of the familial, senile, or essential varieties. N Engl J Med 290: 984–988, 1974

106. Ferro JM, Calhau ES: Treatment of familial essential myoclonus with propranolol. Lancet 2:143, 1977

107. Granville-Grossman KL, Turner P: The effect of propranolol on anxiety. Lancet 1: 788–790, 1966

108. Whitlock FA, Price J: Use of beta adrenergic receptor blocking drugs in psychiatry. Drugs 8:109–124, 1974

109. Editorial: Beta blockers in anxiety and stress. Br Med J 1:415, 1976

110. Jefferson JW: Beta adrenergic blockade in psychiatry. Arch Gen Psychiatr 31:681–691, 1974

111. Atsmon A, Blim I, Steiner M, Latz A, Wijsenbeck H: Further studies with propranolol in psychotic patients. Relation to initial psychiatric state, urinary catecholamines and 3 methoxy 4 hydroxy phenyl glycol. Psycho Pharmacol 27:249–254, 1972

112. Yorkston NJ, Zaki SA, Malik MKU, Morrison RC, and Havard CWH: Propranolol in the control of schizophrenic symptoms. Br Med J 4:633–635, 1974

113. Editorial: New drugs for schizophrenia. Br Med J 4:614–655, 1975

114. Grosz HJ: Narcotic withdrawal symptoms in heroin users treated with propranolol. Lancet 2:564–566, 1972

115. Grosz HJ: Effect of propranolol on active users of heroin. Lancet 2:602, 1973

116. Sellers EM, Degani NC, Silm DH, MacLeod SM: Propranolol-decreased noradrenaline secretion and alcohol withdrawal. Lancet 1:94–95, 1976

117. Boger W, Steinert R, Puliafito C, Pavan-Langston D: Clinical trial comparing timolol ophthalmic solution to pilocarpine in open-angle glaucoma. Am J Ophthalmol 86:8, 1978

118. Zimmerman T, Kaufman H: Timolol: a beta-adrenergic blocking agent for the treatment of glaucoma. Arch Ophthalmol 95:601, 1977

CHAPTER FOUR

Adverse Effects
CHOOSING A β-ADRENOCEPTOR BLOCKER

William H. Frishman, Ralph Silverman,
Joel Strom, and Uri Elkayam

THE adverse effects of β-adrenoreceptor blocking drugs can be divided into two categories: (1) those that result from known pharmacologic consequences of β-adrenoreceptor blockade and (2) other reactions that do not appear to result from β-adrenoreceptor blockade.

Side effects of the first type are widespread because of the ubiquitous nature of the sympathetic nervous system in the control of physiologic and metabolic function. They include asthma, heart failure, hypoglycemia, bradycardia and heart block, intermittent claudication, and Raynaud's phenomenon. The incidence of these adverse effect varies with the type of β-blocker used.

Side effects of the second category are rare. They include an unusual oculomucocutaneous reaction and the possibility of carcinogenesis.

MAJOR CLINICAL TRIALS

There have been extensive clinical trials identifying the nature and frequency of side effects with β-blocking agents. The Boston Collaborative Drug Surveillance Program dealt with propranolol in 800 hospitalized patients, and with practolol in 199 patients.[1] Forrest[2] reported on adverse reactions to oxprenolol among 4400 patients receiving the drug for angina. Two large trials have been carried out with pindolol detailing at length the types and frequency of side effects with this drug.[3,4]

In the Boston Collaborative Drug Surveillance Program, propranolol was used for mixed clinical indications and adverse reactions were reported in 79 patients (9.9 percent). These are summarized in Table 4-1. Ten adverse reactions were considered life-threatening and all appeared to result from impairment of cardiac function. Of the 69 other reactions, 43 also involved interference with cardiac performance but were not life-threatening. The frequency of side effects was independent of the dose used. Reactions were more common among older patients and those with azotemia.

TABLE 4-1 Adverse Reactions to Propranolol
among 800 Hospitalized Medical Patients*

Nature of Reaction	Number of Patients	Percent
Life-threatening		
Shock	5	0.6
Bradycardia and angina	1	0.1
Pulmonary edema	3	0.4
Complete heart block	1	0.1
Total	10	1.3
Nonlife-threatening		
Bradycardia	17	2.1
Hypotension	16	2.0
Congestive heart failure or fluid retention	9	1.1
Gastrointestinal disturbances	9	1.1
CNS disturbances		
(headache, dizziness, fatigue, tinnitus, blurring of vision, paraesthesias, depression)	9	1.1
Bronchospasm	4	0.5
Sensitivity reactions (rash, fever)	3	0.4
2:1 heart block	1	0.1
Elevation in serum phenytoin level	1	0.1
Total	69	8.6
Total with adverse reactions	79	9.9

*With bradycardia in three cases and congestive heart failure in one; with syncope in five cases.

In the same study, of the 199 patients who received practolol, (cardioselective) adverse reactions were reported in 18 (9.0 percent). The nature and frequency of adverse reactions to practolol resembled those of propranolol (Table 4-2). In the studies of oxprenolol[2] and pindolol[3,4] (intrinsic sympathomimetic activity), similar findings were noted.

Overall, the frequency of side effects among the β-blockers is similar. Whether the newer β-blockers with cardioselectivity and/or intrinsic sympathetic activity can alter the nature and severity of these effects will be discussed below. It is important to note, however, that much of our knowledge to date concerning certain side effects is derived either from anecdotal reports or small series of patients.

TABLE 4-2   Adverse Reactions to Practolol
among 199 Hospitalized Medical Patients

Nature of Reaction	Number of Patients	Percent
Life-threatening		
Pulmonary edema	1	0.5
Complete heart block, bradycardia, and shock	1	0.5
Second degree heart block and hypotension	1	0.5
Total	3	1.5
Nonlife-Threatening		
Congestive heart failure	3	1.5
Bradycardia	4	2.0
CNS disturbances (dizziness, confusion)	3	1.5
Sensitivity reactions (rash)	2	1.0
Hypotension	1	0.5
Gastrointestinal disturbances	1	0.5
Dyspnea	1	0.5
Total	15	7.5
Total with adverse reactions	18	9.0

ADVERSE CARDIAC EFFECTS
RELATED TO β-ADRENOCEPTOR BLOCKADE

CARDIAC FAILURE

There are several circumstances in which blockade of β-receptors may cause congestive heart failure: (1) in an enlarged heart with impaired myocardial function where excessive sympathetic drive is essential to maintain it on a compensated Starling curve; and (2) if the stroke volume is restricted and tachycardia is needed to maintain cardiac output.

Considering the factors noted above, *any* β-blocking drug may be associated with the development of heart failure. Furthermore, it is possible that an important component of heart failure may be accounted for by increases in peripheral resistance produced by nonselective agents (e.g., propranolol, timolol, sotalol).[6] Practolol is less likely to produce cardiac decompensation; the hemodynamic effects of newer cardioselective agents in patients with myocardial dysfunction has yet to be determined.

It has been claimed that β-blockers with intrinsic sympathomimetic activity are less likely to precipitate heart failure, but there have been no in vivo studies to support this contention and it has been shown that these drugs can precipitate heart failure.[7] In dog-transplanted denervated heart preparations, β-blockers with intrinsic sympathomimetic activity, have a positive rather than a negative inotropic effect.[8] The clinical significance of this effect is uncertain.

In patients with impaired myocardial function who need β-blocking agents, digitalis and diuretics may be used preferably with drugs having cardioselectivity or intrinsic sympathomimetic activity.

ATRIOVENTRICULAR CONDUCTION DELAY AND SINUS NODE DYSFUNCTION

Slowing of the resting heart rate is a normal response to treatment with a β-blocking drug without intrinsic sympathomimetic activity. Healthy individuals can sustain a heart rate of 50 without disability, unless there is clinical evidence for heart failure.[5] Drugs with intrinsic sympathomimetic activity do not lower the resting heart rate to the same degree as propranolol, however, all β-blocking drugs are contraindicated (unless an artificial pacemaker is present) in patients with the "sick sinus syndrome."[9]

If there is a partial or complete atrioventricular conduction defect, use of a β-blocking drug may lead to a serious bradyarrhythmia.[5] The risk of atrioventricular impairment is not the same with all β-blockers. Giudicelli et al.[10] showed that in dogs β-blockade and not membrane-stabilizing activity is responsible for atrioventricular conduction impairment. Compounds, like pindolol or practolol, which have intrinsic sympathomimetic activity in dosages producing β-blockade, do not impair atrioventricular conduction.

β-ADRENOCEPTOR BLOCKER WITHDRAWAL

Following the abrupt cessation of β-blocker therapy after chronic administration, exacerbation of angina pectoris and, in some cases, acute myocardial infarction have been reported.[11-13]

Two double-blind randomized trials confirmed the reality of a propranolol withdrawal syndrome.[12-13] The mechanism for the propranolol withdrawal effect is unclear and may be related to the multifactorial actions of the drug. Reduced exercise tolerance following abrupt withdrawal of chronic propranolol therapy, in patients with angina pectoris, may be due to loss of sympathetic blockade of cardiovascular function resulting in an acute increase in myocardial oxygen demands. Our group demonstrated that abrupt propranolol withdrawal can possibly harm some patients with angina pectoris by causing rebound platelet hyperaggregability associated with increased anginal frequency, decreased exercise tolerance, and possible compromise of coronary blood flow.[13]

A "rebound" effect has not been well-defined with the other β-blocking agents. It seems that discontinuation of β-blocker therapy should be done gradually and cautiously in patients with ischemic heart disease, however.

ADVERSE NONCARDIAC SIDE EFFECTS RELATED TO β-ADRENORECEPTOR BLOCKADE

EFFECT ON VENTILATORY FUNCTION

The bronchodilator effects of catecholamines on the bronchial β-adrenoreceptors (β_2) are prevented by β-blockade with nonselective agents (e.g., propranolol).[14] Comparative studies have shown, however, that compounds with intrinsic sympathomimetic activity and/or cardioselectivity are less likely to increase airway resistance in asthmatics than propranolol.[15-17] Cardioselectivity is not absolute, and with higher doses may be lost as has been shown with practolol. Since β_1 selectivity is not absolute, a β_2 stimulating agent can be helpful when used concomitantly in patients with bronchospastic disease.[18] In general, however, all β-blockers should be avoided in patients with active bronchospastic disease.

PERIPHERAL VASCULAR EFFECTS (RAYNAUD'S PHENOMENON)

Cold extremities and absent pulses have been described to occur more frequently in patients receiving β-blockers for hypertension, compared with methyldopa.[19] Among the β-blockers the incidence was highest with propranolol and lower with drugs having cardioselectivity or intrinsic sympathomimetic activity. In some instances, vascular compromise has been severe enough to cause cyanosis and impending gangrene.[20] This is due to the reduction in cardiac output and blockade of β-adrenergic mediated skeletal muscle vasodilation, resulting in unopposed α-adrenoceptor vasoconstriction.[21] β-Blocking drugs with cardioselectivity or intrinsic sympathetic activity will not affect peripheral vessels to the same degree as propranolol.

Raynaud's phenomenon is one of the more common side effects of propranolol treatment.[22,23] It is more troublesome with propranolol than practolol, probably due to the β_2-blocking properties of propranolol.

Patients with peripheral vascular disease who suffer from intermittent claudication often report worsening of the claudication when treated with β-blocking drugs.[24,25] Whether drugs with cardioselectivity in intrinsic sympathomimetic activity can protect against this side effect has yet to be determined.

HYPOGLYCEMIA AND HYPERGLYCEMIA

Several authors have described severe hypoglycemic reactions during therapy with β-adrenergic blocking drugs.[26,27] Some of the patients affected were insulin-dependent diabetics, while others were nondiabetic. Studies of resting normal volunteers have demonstrated that propranolol produces no alteration in blood glucose values[28] although the hyperglycemic response to exercise is blunted.

In man, mobilization of muscle glycogen is a β-receptor-mediated function (β_2-mediated), while mobilization of liver glycogen depends on α-receptor stimulation.[29,30] As a result, β-receptor blocking drugs (especially nonselective β-blockers) may retard recovery from insulin induced hypoglycemia. In humans, Abramson et al.[26] showed that propranolol delayed the return of blood glucose values to normal after insulin-induced hypoglycemia.

Likewise, if liver glycogen is reduced by fasting or illness, the concomitant administration of β-blocking drugs may prolong recovery from hypoglycemia since alternative stores cannot be mobilized.[31]

There is also a marked diminution in the manifestations of sympathetic discharge associated with hypoglycemia.[32] These findings suggest that propranolol (noncardioselective) interferes with compensatory responses to hypoglycemia and can mask certain "warning signs" of this condition. This enhancement of insulin induced-hypoglycemia may be less with cardioselective agents (where there is no blocking effect on β_2-receptors) and agents with intrinsic sympathomimetic activity (which may stimulate β_2-receptors).[33]

CENTRAL NERVOUS SYSTEM EFFECTS

Dreams, hallucinations, insomnia, and depression can occur during therapy with the β-blockers.[22] These symptoms are evidence of drug entry into the central nervous system (CNS) and are especially common with the highly lipid-soluble β-blockers (propranolol, alprenolol) which presumably penetrate the CNS better. Vivid dreams may also occur with other agents (practolol, pindolol), a lesser penetration into the CNS notwithstanding.

Severe depression has been described with propranolol therapy, especially in patients receiving high doses over long periods of time. Oxprenolol, which has partial agonist activity, was found to have a stimulant rather than a depressant central nervous system action; but occasionally, it too can cause depression.[34]

Clinical pharmacologic studies have generally supported the view that β-blockers do not have any marked sedative effect. No such action could be detected for propranolol, sotalol, oxprenolol, or atenolol.[35]

SKELETAL MUSCLE EFFECTS

In vitro studies demonstrate that propranolol can produce neuromuscular blockade.[1] The direct actions of epinephrine on skeletal muscle are mediated probably through β_2-receptors and tremor is the most common side effect of β_2-stimulating drugs. Propranolol has been shown to attenuate the angle jerk and a prolonged curarelike effect has been described in one patient.[36] Whether the cardioselective β-blockers have similar effects remains to be determined.

Muscle cramps can occur also with pindolol[22] and have been described with practolol and propranolol.[37] The etiology of this side effect is unknown.

MISCELLANEOUS SIDE EFFECTS

Diarrhea, nausea, gastric pain, constipation and flatulence have been seen occasionally with all β-blockers (2 to 11 percent of patients).

Hematalogic reactions are rare: rare cases of purpura,[38] and agranulocytosis[39] have been described with propranolol.

A devastating blood pressure rebound effect has been described in patients who discontinued clonidine while being treated with nonselective β-blocking agents. The mechanism for this may be related to an increase in peripheral resistance.[40,41] Whether cardioselective β-blockers have similar effects following clonidine withdrawal remains to be determined.

Increase in patient weight may occur: Bengtsson[42] noted an average 1-kg weight increment in patients taking alprenolol. A similar weight gain in patients has also been noted with propranolol,[43] pindolol,[44] and oxprenolol. The mechanism of this weight gain has not been elucidated, however, treatment with diuretic agents will commonly relieve it.

ADVERSE EFFECTS UNRELATED TO β-ADRENOCEPTOR BLOCKADE

OCULOMUCOCUTANEOUS SYNDROME

A characteristic immune reaction — the oculomucocutaneous syndrome — affecting singly or in combination eyes, mucous and serous membranes, and the skin, often in association with a positive antinuclear factor, has been reported in patients treated with practolol, and has lead to the curtailment of its use.[45,46] Close attention has been focused on this syndrome because of fears that other β-adrenoreceptor blocking drugs may be associated with this syndrome.

The main features in this syndrome in 439 patients reviewed by Nichols[5] were as follows:

Eye. A gritty feeling in the eye may occur which can progress to a pan-conjunctivitis, keratitis, and pannus formation. In Nichol's series, 18 patients manifested severe eye changes, 112 had corneal damage without loss of sight, and 146 had eye changes without corneal involvement. The average time to develop this syndrome was 23 months after initiating treatment.

Skin. The skin changes usually begin with a pruritic rash involving the palms and the soles of the feet. Thickened plaques which resemble psoriasis may appear. Immunofluorescent studies have revealed granular deposits at the dermalectodermal junction in some cases.[47]

Ear. Deafness with serious otitis media has been reported in some patients receiving practolol.

SCLEROSING PERITONITIS

Thirty-three patients with this syndrome were included in Nichol's report. Patients may present with colicky abdominal pain or with an abdominal mass. This condition may progress in spite of withdrawal of the drug and first develop up to a year after the discontinuation of practolol. The peritoneum becomes covered with a film of white fibrous tissue with thicker plaques.[48] The natural history of the condition is unknown and the diagnosis has usually been made at laparotomy or autopsy. Most patients appear to improve with time after cessation of treatment. The mean time to diagnosis of sclerosing peritonitis after starting practolol was 37 months.

As with sclerosing peritonitis, many of the other practolol reactions are reversible by withdrawal of the drug, together with topical corticosteroids, artifical tear solutions, antibiotic eye drops, and oral corticosteroids.

An important consideration is whether the practolol reaction is specific for practolol or is the direct and specific result of pharmacologically induced changes by β-blockade.[49] There have been few convincing published reports of the oculomucocutaneous reaction with oxprenolol[50, 51] and propranolol.[52, 53] For the most part, these were specific ocular symptoms and signs without any real evidence to suggest they might reflect an adverse effect to any drug.[54]

In view of the extensive and long use of both oxprenolol and propranolol, these reactions, even if drug induced, are exceedingly rare. There is need, however, for vigilance for these reactions during therapy with the newer β-blockers.

CARCINOGENICITY

Pronethanol, the first β-adrenoceptor blocking drug to achieve wide use, was withdrawn by its manufacturers because it caused thymic tumors and lymphosarcomata in mice, although it did not do so in rats or dogs.[55] The doses used to produce these tumors were 10 times the maximum therapeutic concentration.

Recently, tolamolol and pamatolol, two cardioselective β-adrenoreceptor blocking drugs, were withdrawn from clinical trials because they caused mammary tumors in mice and rats at high doses.[56] Other β-blockers, alprenolol and practolol, have given some indication of tumorigenicity in rodents.[56]

The relevance of these findings to causation of tumors in man is difficult to evaluate. The doses were high and the relationship between malignant tumors in animals and man is not defined. A disturbing aspect has been the suggestion that this might be a pharmacologic property of β-adrenoceptor antagonism rather than carcinogenicity by other mechanism. Against the β-blocker theory of carcinogenesis is the fact that many β-blocking drugs (including many described in this series) have passed successfully stringent carcinogenicity testing in animals.

HOW TO CHOOSE A β-BLOCKER

The various β-blocking compounds given in adequate dosage have comparable, antihypertensive, antiarrhythmic, and antianginal effects. Therefore the β-blocking drug of choice in an individual patient is determined by the pharmacological and pharmacokinetic differences between the drugs in conjunction with the other medical conditions the patient might have (Table 4-3).

TABLE 4-3   Clinical Situations that would Influence the Choice of a β-Blocking Drug

Condition	Choice of β-Blocker
Asthma, chronic bronchitis with bronchospasm	Avoid all β-blockers if possible; however small doses of cardioselective β-blockers (e.g., acebutolol, atenolol, metoprolol) can be used. Cardioselectivity is lost with higher doses. Drugs with partial agonist activity (e.g., pindolol, alprenolol) can also be used.
Congestive heart failure	Drugs with partial agonist activity might have an advantage, although β-blockers are usually contraindicated.
Angina	In patients with angina at low heart rates, drugs with partial agonist activity probably contraindicated. Patients with angina at high heart rates but who have resting bradycardia might benefit from a drug with partial agonist activity.
Atrioventricular conduction defects	β-Blockers generally contraindicated but drugs with partial agonist activity can be tried with caution.

(continued)

TABLE 4-3   (cont.)

Condition	Choice of β-Blocker
Bradycardia	β-Blockers with partial agonist activity have less pulse slowing effect and are preferable.
Raynaud's phenomenon, intermittent claudication, cold extremities	Cardioselective agents and those with partial agonist activity might have an advantage.
Depression	Avoid propranolol. Substitute a β-blocker with partial agonist activity.
Diabetes mellitus	Cardioselective agents preferable.
Thyrotoxicosis	All agents with control symptoms but agents without partial agonist activity are preferred.
Pheochromocytoma	Avoid all β-blockers unless an alpha-blocker is given.
Renal failure	Use reduced doses of compounds largely eliminated by renal mechanisms (sotalol, atenolol) and of those drugs whose bioavailability is increased in uremia (propranolol, alprenolol). Also consider possible accumulation of active metabolites (alprenolol, propranolol).
Insulin and sulphonylurea use	Danger of hypoglycemia. Possibly less using drugs with cardioselectivity.
Clonidine	Avoid sotalol (other nonselective β-blockers). Severe rebound effect with clonidine withdrawal.
Oculomucocutaneous syndrome	Stop drug. Substitute any other β-blocker.

REFERENCES

1. Greenblatt DJ, Koch-Weser J: Clinical toxicity of propranolol and practolol. A report from the Boston Collaborative Drug Surveillance Program. In Avery G (ed): Cardiovascular Drugs, Vol. II. Baltimore, University Park Press, 1978, pp 179–195
2. Forrest WA: A monitored release study: a clinical trial of oxprenolol in general practice. Practitioner 208:412–416, 1972
3. Collins IS, King IW: Pindolol (Visken LB 46), a new treatment for hypertension: report of a multicentric open study. Curr Ther Res 14:185–194, 1972
4. Morgan TO, Louis WJ, Dawborn JK, Doyle AE: The use of prindolol (Visken) in the treatment of hypertension. Med J Aust 2:309–312, 1972
5. Conolly ME, Kersting F, Dollery CT: The clinical pharmacology of beta-adrenoceptor-blocking drugs. Prog Card Dis 19:203–234, 1976
6. Vaughan Williams EM, Baywell EE, Singh BN: Cardiospecificity of beta-receptor

blockade. A comparison of the relative potencies on cardiac and peripheral vascular beta-adrenoceptors of propranolol, of practolol and its ortho-substituted isomer and of oxprenolol and its para-substituted isomer. Cardiovasc Res 7:226–240, 1973

7. Fitzgerald JD: Perspectives in adrenergic beta-receptor blockade. Clin Pharm Ther 10: 292–306, 1969

8. Nayler WG: The effect of beta-adrenergic receptor blocking drugs on myocardial function: an explanation of the subcellular level. In Simpson F (ed): Ciba Symposium Beta-Adrenergic Receptor Blocking Drugs Sydney, Australasian Drug Information Services, 1970, pp 1–12

9. Singh BN, Jewitt DE: β-adrenoceptor blocking drugs in cardiac arrhythmias. In Avery G (ed): Cardiovascular Drugs Vol. II. Baltimore, University Park Press, 1978, pp 119–159

10. Giudicelli JF, Lhoste F, Bossier JR: β-adrenergic blockade and atrio-ventricular conduction impairment. Eur J Pharmacol 31:216–225, 1975

11. Alderman EL, Coltart DJ, Wettach GE, Harrison DC: Coronary artery syndromes after sudden propranolol withdrawal. Ann Intern Med 81:925–927, 1974

12. Miller RR, Olson HG, Amsterdam EA, Mason DT: Propranolol withdrawal rebound phenomenon: exacerbation of coronary events after abrupt cessation of anti-anginal therapy. N En J Med 293:416–418, 1975

13. Frishman WH, Christodoulou J, Weksler B, et al.: Abrupt propranolol withdrawal in angina pectoris: Effects on platelet aggregation and exercise tolerance. Am Heart J 95:169–179, 1978

14. Dunlop D, Shanks RG: Selective blockade of adrenoceptive beta receptors in the heart. Br J Pharmacol Chemother 32:201–218, 1968

15. Beumer HM, Hardonk HJ: Effects of beta-adrenergic blocking drugs on ventilatory failure in asthmatics. Eur J Clin Pharmacol 5:77–80, 1972–1973

16. Singh BN, Whitlock RML, Combes RH, Williams FH, Harris EA: Effects of cardioselective β-adrenoceptor blockade on specific airways resistance in normal subjects and in patients with bronchial asthma. Clin Pharmacol Ther 19:493–501, 1976

17. Skinner C, Gaddu J, Palmer KNV: Comparison of effects of metoprolol and propranolol on asthmatic airway obstruction. Br Med J 1:504, 1976

18. Formgren H, Eriksson ME: Effects of practolol in combination with terbutaline in the treatment of hypertension and arrhythmias in asthmatic patients. Scand J Respir Dis (Suppl) 56:217–222, 1975

19. Waal-Manning HJ: Hypertension: Which Beta-Blocker. Drugs 12:412–441, 1976

20. Frolich ED, Tarazi RC, Dustan HP: Peripheral arterial insufficiency: a complication of beta adrenergic blocking therapy. JAMA 208:2471–2472, 1969

21. Lundvall J, Järhult J: Beta adrenergic dilator component of the sympathetic vascular response in skeletal muscle. Acta Physiol Scand 96:180–192, 1976

22. Simpson FO: β-Adrenergic receptor blocking drugs in hypertension. Drugs 7:85–105, 1974

23. Zacharias FJ, Cowen KJ, Prestt J, Vickers J, Wall BG: Propranolol in hypertension: A study of long term therapy. 1964–1970 Am Heart J 83:755–761, 1972

24. George CF: Beta-receptor blocking agents. Prescriber's Journal 14:93–98, 1974

25. Rodger JC, Sheldon CD, Lerski RA, Livingston WR: Intermittent claudication complicating beta-blockade. Br Med J 1:1125, 1976

26. Abramson EA, Arky RA, Woeber KA: Effects of propranolol on the hormonal and metabolic responses to insulin induced hypoglycemia. Lancet 2:1386-1388, 1966

27. Reveno WS, Rosenbaum H: Propranolol hypoglycemia. Lancet 1:920, 1968

28. Allison SP, Chamberlain MI, Miller JE: Effects of propranolol on blood sugar, insulin, and free fatty acids. Diabetologia 5:339-342, 1969

29. Porte D: Sympathetic regulation of insulin secretion. Its relation to diabetes mellitus. Arch Intern Med 183:252, 1969

30. Antonis A, Clark ML, Hodge RL, et al.: Receptor mechanisms in the hyperglycaemic response to adrenaline in man. Lancet 1:1135-1137, 1967

31. Dollery CT, Paterson JW, Conolly ME: Clinical pharmacology of beta blocking drugs. Clin Pharmacol Ther 10:765-799, 1969

32. Lloyd-Mostyn RH, Oram S: Modification by propranolol of cardiovascular effects of induced hypoglycaemia. Lancet 2:1213-1215, 1975

33. Deacon SP, Barnett D: Comparison of atenolol and propranolol during insulin-induced hypoglycaemia. Br Med J 2:7-9, 1976

34. Waal H: Propranolol-induced depression. Br Med J 2:50, 1967

35. Bayliss PFC, Duncan SM: The effects of atenolol (Tenormin) and methyldopa on simple tests of central nervous function. Br J Clin Pharmacol 2:527-531, 1975

36. Rozen MS, Whan FM: Prolonged curarization associated with propranolol. Med J Aust 1:467-468, 1972

37. Greenblatt DJ, Koch-Weser J: Adverse reactions to β-adrenergic receptor blocking drugs: A report from the Boston Collaborative Drug Surveillance Program. Drugs 7: 118-129, 1974

38. Stephens SA: Unwanted effects of propranolol. Am J Cardiol 18:463-472, 1966

39. Nawabi IU, Ritz ND: Agranulocytosis due to propranolol. JAMA 223:1376-1377, 1973

40. Bailey R, Neale TJ: Rapid clonidine withdrawal with blood pressure overshoot exaggerated by beta blockade. Br Med J 1:942-943, 1976

41. Cairns SA, Marshall AJ: Clonidine withdrawal. Lancet 1:368, 1976

42. Bengtsson C: Comparison between alprenolol and chlorthalidone as anti-hypertensive agents. Acta Med Scand 191:433-439, 1972

43. Seedat YK, Stewart-Wynne E: Clinical experiences with prindolol (Visken) in the therapy of hypertension. South Afr Med J 46:1524-1526, 1972

44. Waal-Manning HJ, Simpson FO: Pindolol: a comparison with other anti-hypertensive drugs and a double-blind placebo trial. Aust NZ Med J 80:151-157, 1974

45. Wright P: Untoward effect associated with practolol administration. Oculomucocutaneous syndrome. Br Med J 1:595-598, 1975

46. Waal-Manning H: Problems with practolol. Drugs 10:336-341, 1975

47. Felix RH, Ive FA, Dahl MCG: Cutaneous and ocular reactions to practolol. Br Med J 4: 321-324, 1974

48. Windsor WP, Durrein F, Dyer NH: Fibrinous peritonitis: A complication of practolol therapy. Br Med J 2:68, 1975

49. Gaylarde PM, Sukany I: Side effects of practolol. Br Med J 2:435-438, 1975

50. Holt PJA, Waddington E: Oculocutaneous reaction to oxprenolol. Br Med J 2: 539-540, 1975

51. Knapp MS, Gallaway HR, Clayden JR: Ocular reactions to beta blockers. Br Med J 2: 557, 1975

52. Cubey RB, Taylor SH: Ocular reaction to propranolol and resolution on continued treatment with a different beta blocking drug. Br Med J 4:327–328, 1975
53. Harty RP: Sclerosing peritonitis and propranolol. Arch Intern Med 138:1424, 1978
54. Wright P: Ocular reactions to beta-blocking drugs. Br Med J: 577, 1975
55. Paget GE: Carcinogenic actions of pronethalol. Br Med J 2:1266–1277, 1963
56. Status Report on Beta-Blockers. FDA Drug Bulletin 8:13, 1978

CHAPTER FIVE

Self-Poisoning with β-Adrenoceptor Blocking Drugs
RECOGNITION AND MANAGEMENT

William H. Frishman, Harold Jacob,
Edward Eisenberg, and Hillel Ribner

B ETA-ADRENOCEPTOR blocking drugs are now widely prescribed for a multitude of indications in clinical medicine.[1] They are extensively used either alone, or in combination with other agents to treat cardiac arrhythmias of ventricular or supraventricular origin, angina pectoris, obstructive cardiomyopathies, essential hypertension, and thyrotoxicosis.[2] β-Adrenoceptor blocking drugs may also be of benefit in some patients with hyperkinetic heart syndromes, migraine headache, essential tremor, anxiety, psychoses, acne vulgaris, alcohol and narcotic withdrawal, and septic shock.[1,2]

The β-adrenoceptor blocking drugs have many associated adverse effects when used in the therapeutic dose range, which were described in Chapter 4.[3] With the growing application of these drugs in clinical practice, cases of attempted suicide and accidental overdosage are being reported. The clinical manifestations of massive intoxication in humans have not been well-appreciated. Moreover, the management of patients with overdosage is a subject of controversy. Variations in the pharmacologic properties of the different β-adrenoceptor blockers (cardioselectivity, partial agonist effect) affect their therapeutic actions and adverse effects.[2-5] These individual differences may influence the clinical features of serious overdosage.

In this chapter we will review: (1) our own experiences in four patients with propranolol intoxication; (2) the world experience with β-adrenoceptor blocking drug overdosage; (3) the currently recommended therapeutic modalities for this problem.

CASE REPORTS

Four cases of massive propranolol intoxication seen at our institution are
described below. Data from these patients are summarized in Table 5-1.

TABLE 5-1.   Summary of Four Patients with Propranolol Overdosage Treated
at the Bronx Municipal Hospital Center

	No. 1	No. 2	No. 3	No. 4
Age	17	25	19	59
Sex	F	F	F	M
Plasma level (ng/ml)	449*	2300	2800	1800
Estimated ingestion (mg)	1200–1600	?	1600	2000
Heart rate (beats/min)	50	116→50	80→50	50
Blood pressure (mm Hg)	Unobtainable	150/100→ Unobtainable	130/80→90/60	120/70
Preantidote:				
Level of consciousness	Comatose	Alert/agitated	Comatose	Semidelirious
Convulsions	Yes	Yes	Yes	No
Congestive heart failure	No	No	No	Yes
Bronchospasm	No	No	No	No
Blood sugar (mg/dl)	136	207	135	150
ECG findings	Regular rhythm, 1st degree heart block, IVCD†	NSR, IVCD	Regular rhythm, 1st degree heart block, IVCD	Regular rhythm, 1st degree heart block, IVCD
Treatment	Diazepam, epinephrine	Atropine, phenobarbital isoproterenol, glucagon, dopamine	Diazepam, atropine, glucagon, isoproterenol	Pacemaker, oxygen, atropine, glucagon, isoproterenol

*Obtained after 24 hours admission.
†Intraventricular conduction defect

CASE 1.   A 17-year-old, previously healthy female, was brought to the
emergency room 2 hours after ingesting 30 to 40 of her mother's 40-mg propranolol (Inderal) tablets (1200 to 1600 mg) in a suicide attempt. Within 90
minutes of ingestion, she had become stuporous and experienced generalized seizures lasting several minutes. She was comatose, with only avoid-

ance responses to painful stimuli on arrival at the hospital. Blood pressure was unobtainable, heart rate 50 per minute, and respiratory rate 20 per minute with shallow chest excursions. Pupils were 4 mm, equal, and reactive to light. There were rhonchi at both bases. The extremities were cool but not cyanotic; tendon reflexes were moderately active and symmetrical. Minutes after arriving at the hospital the patient had a generalized tonic-clonic seizure which responded promptly to 5 mg of intravenous diazepam. She was then given two doses of 0.06 mg of epinephrine intravenously resulting in an increase of the heart rate to 70 per minute and blood pressure to 90/50 mm Hg. At the time of admission serum sodium concentration was 138 mEq per liter, potassium 4.5 mEq per liter, calcium 8.1 mg per dl, bicarbonate 21 mEq per liter, chloride 100 mEq per liter, and glucose 136 mg per dl. Arterial pH was 7.30, PCO_2 26 mm Hg, and PO_2 mm Hg. Routine toxicologic screening showed the presence of a barbiturate in the first of two specimens of gastric contents; however, urine screening was negative. The patient had no prior history of seizures or cardiovascular disease. Her level of consciousness improved over the next several hours and the day after admission she was alert and oriented with a completely normal neurologic exam. Serum propranolol levels were not drawn immediately on arrival, but 24 hours later the serum propranolol measured spectrofluorometrically was 449 ng per ml decreasing to 19 ng per ml at 48 hours after admission, and to nondetectable levels at 96 hours. An ECG taken upon admission showed regular sinus rhythm, first degree heart block, and an intraventricular conduction defect. Twenty-four hours later the ECG was normal. An EEG performed on the 8th hospital day was normal.

CASE 2. A 25-year-old woman came to the Bronx Municipal Hospital Emergency Room 30 minutes after ingesting "two handfuls" of 40-mg propranolol (Inderal) tablets in a suicide attempt. She was alert and agitated, had a pulse of 116 per minute and a blood pressure of 150/100. The patient received 30 ml of Ipecac syrup and several minutes later she vomited green pill fragments. Subsequently, she suffered a grand mal seizure. At that point her blood pressure was unobtainable and her pulse 50 per minute. The patient was given 1 mg of atropine, 2 mg of isoproterenol, and 4 mg of glucagon intravenously, and subsequently was begun on continuous infusions of isoproterenol, glucagon, and dopamine with a resultant increase in her pulse to 80 per minute and blood pressure to 80/50 mm Hg. Despite injection of phenobarbital, 240 mg intravenously, she then experienced two more generalized seizures, each lasting only seconds. Physical exam shortly thereafter was remarkable for a lethargic but arousable woman whose pupils were each 6 mm and reactive to light. The remainder of the examination was unremarkable. At the time of admission serum sodium concentration was 139 mEq per liter, potassium 3.5 mEq per liter, bicarbonate 15 mEq per liter, calcium 9.7 mg per dl, chloride 100 mEq per liter, and glucose 207 mg per dl. Arterial blood pH was 7.41, PCO_2 20 mm Hg and PO_2 75 mm Hg. Toxicologic screening of the urine was negative for any drugs. Serum propranolol levels done spectroflurometrically were 2300 ng per ml on admission, 800 ng per ml 5 hours later, and 300 ng per ml 24 hours later. An ECG (Fig. 5-1) taken upon admission revealed normal sinus rhythm with a QRS duration of 0.12 seconds. Twenty-four hours after admission the ECG was normal. The patient made an uneventful recovery.

CASE 3. A 19-year-old female with a history of paroxysmal atrial tachycardia ingested 80 20-mg tablets of propranolol in a suicide attempt, and was brought to the emergency room one hour later in a semiconscious state. She had a pulse rate of 80 and a blood pressure of 130/80 mm Hg. A nasogastric tube was inserted for gastric lavage, with recovery of pill fragments, and activated charcoal was given. Fifteen minutes later she became delerious then unresponsive and experienced a grand mal seizure. Her blood pressure at the time was 90/60 mm Hg and her heart rate 50 per minute. The patient was treated with 1 mg of intravenous atropine and 2 mg of intravenous isoproterenol with no response in heart rate and blood pressure. Intravenous diazepam was given after which the seizures stopped. An infusion of isoproterenol and glucagon were begun which resulted in an increase in her blood pressure to 110/60 mm Hg and her pulse to 70 per minute. Physical exam revealed a lethargic but arousable woman with reactive pupils. Chest and cardiac examinations were unremarkable. Her admission serum sodium was 139 mEq per liter, potassium 3.8 mEq per liter, bicarbonate 17 mEq per liter, calcium 9.4 mg per dl, chloride 99 mEq per liter, and glucose 135 mg per dl. Toxicologic screening was negative for drugs. An initial plasma propranolol level was 2800 ng per ml, 1100 ng per ml, five hours later, and 270 ng per ml 24 hours later. An ECG taken upon admission demonstrated first degree heart block with a PR interval of 0.24 seconds and a QRS duration of 0.10 seconds. Twelve hours later her ECG was normal with a QRS duration of 0.06 seconds. Her chest roentgenogram upon admission showed no evidence of left ventricular dilation or pulmonary congestion. Subsequent neurologic examinations were unremarkable, and the patient made an uneventful recovery.

CASE 4. A 59-year-old male with long-standing hypertension but no other known cardiac disease ingested approximately 50 of his 40-mg propranolol tablets in a suicide attempt. He was brought to the emergency room in acute pulmonary edema, cyanotic, and semidelerious. Upon arrival in the Emergency Room, he was found to have a blood pressure of 120/70 mm Hg and a weak pulse at a rate of 50 per minute. He was treated with oxygen, rotating tourniquets, and 80 mg of intravenous furosemide. The chest ro-

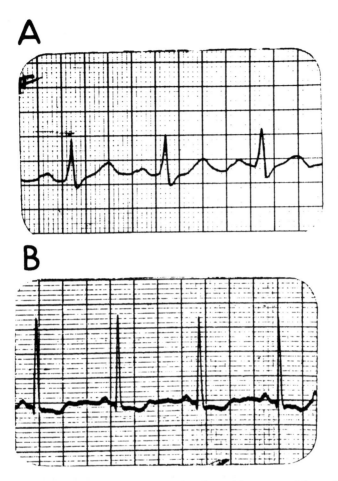

Figure 5-1. Electrocardiogram (lead III) of patient with propranolol overdose (Case #1). **A.** The upper tracing was taken at the time of hospital admission and shows regular sinus rhythm, 1st degree heart block (prolonged PR interval), and an intraventricular conduction defect. **B.** The lower tracing (lead III) taken 24 hours later with another electrocardiograph shows nonspecific ST segment depression and normalization of conduction intervals.

entgenogram revealed fluffy alveolar infiltrates and cardiomegaly and the ECG demonstrated first degree heart block (PR interval of 0.24 seconds) and a heart rate of 50 per minute. There was QRS widening of 0.11 seconds.

The patient received 1 mg of IV atropine and 1 mg isoproterenol with no increment in heart rate. A transvenous pacemaker was inserted with the rate set at 70 per minute, and 10 mg of glucagon were injected intravenously. The patient responded within 10 to 15 minutes with improvement in his cardiovascular status and was maintained on a isoproterenol and glucagon intravenous infusion for 8 hours. The pacemaker was removed after 24 hours. The subsequent ECG revealed a heart rate of 76 per minute with normal PR and QRS durations. A plasma propranolol level done at the time of admission was 1800 ng per ml. An echocardiogram performed 72 hours after admission revealed left ventricular hypertrophy and a slightly diminished ejection fraction. The patient was discharged, following psychi-atric evaluation, with no further cardiac disorder.

COMMENT

These four cases of propranolol self-poisoning reveal many of the features of massive β-adrenoceptor blocker intoxication: hypotension, bradycardia, prolonged atrioventricular conduction times.[6] An unusual feature was that three of the patients had grand mal seizure activity. In only one previous instance of massive overdosage with propranolol have generalized seizures been described.[7] Drug-induced hypoglycemia and other metabolic causes of seizures were ruled out. Although cerebral hypoperfusion may have contributed, the second and third patient suffered convulsions despite an adequate blood pressure. The seizures were responsive to intravenous diazepam in two patients, and unresponsive to phenobarbital in one patient. After recovery in all patients, there was no evidence of neurologic disease.

All four patients had significant changes in their levels of consciousness ranging from frank coma to delerium. Propranolol is a β-adrenoceptor blocking agent which is not cardioselective and has membrane depressant action (quinidine or local anesthetic property).[4] The drug is extremely lipid soluble and rapidly crosses the blood–brain barrier to concentrate in brain tissue. The membrane depressant effect of propranolol is not important in the usual therapeutic dose range,[8] however, it might become important with massive intoxications. The seizures and change in mental status may be similar to effects seen with lidocaine, another lipophilic local anesthetic drug.[9]

Another unusual presentation was the widening of the QRS complex of the electrocardiogram, evidence of an intraventricular conduction defect. This finding is not a feature of the propranolol effect in usual therapeutic doses.[2] It may be a result of the "quinidine" or membrane depressant effect of propranolol which is seen with massive doses.[8]

No patient had definite evidence of bronchospasm or developed hypoglycemia. Patient 4 developed acute pulmonary edema following a 2-gm propranolol ingestion. Higher doses have been given to patients with normal hearts over 24 hours without evidence of left ventricular decompensation.[10] On the other hand, patients with occult myocardopathy have gone into pulmonary edema with as little as 40 mg of propranolol. It may be that patient 4 had an occult hypertensive cardiomyopathy which only manifested itself after the self-poisoning episode.

All patients responded to therapy and recovered from their overdosage without sequelae.

REVIEW OF THE WORLD EXPERIENCE WITH β-ADRENOCEPTOR BLOCKER SELF-POISONING

Variations in pharmacologic properties of the different β-adrenoceptor blocking agents (Table 5-2) affect their therapeutic action and predictable side effects.[2-5,11,12] These differences may influence the clinical presentation of massive overdosage. The reported cases of β-adrenoceptor self-poisoning are reviewed below and summarized in Table 5-3.

Acebutolol. (cardioselective, partial agonist-activity, membrane depressant). There have been no reports of self-poisoning with acebutolol to date.

Alprenolol. (noncardioselective, partial agonist activity, membrane depressant). One fatal case of alprenolol self-poisoning has been reported in a 32-year-old female, who ingested 12.8 gm of drug (approximately 64 200-mg tablets).[13] She presented with hypotension, coma, and had a respiratory arrest. Despite the supportive measures, the patient eventually developed asystole and died. Her postmortem alprenolol blood level was 1300 ng per ml.

Atenolol. (cardioselective, no partial agonist activity or membrane depressant effects). A 24-year-old female who was receiving atenolol for treatment of hypertension ingested 1200 mg of drug six times greater than the therapeutic dose in a suicide attempt.[14] She was admitted to the hospital 2 to 3 hours later in good condition. Her pulse rate was 80 beats per minute with a recumbent blood pressure of 150/110 mm Hg. There were no signs of cardiac decompensation and the ECG was normal. She was closely monitored over the ensuing days during which time her pulse rate varied between 66 to 60 beats per minute in sinus rhythm. Her blood pressure was 190/120 mm Hg 5 days after ingestion. The clinical course was uncomplicated.

Metoprolol. (cardioselective, no partial agonist activity, weak membrane depressant activity). Two cases of nonfatal metoprolol intoxication have been reported:

1. A 19-year-old male was admitted to the hospital after having ingested 200 50 mg tablets (10,000 mg).[15] Upon arrival at the hospital he was con-

TABLE 5-2. Summary of Pharmacologic Properties of β-Adrenoceptor Blocking Drugs

Drug	Cardio-selectivity	Partial Agonist Activity	Membrane Stabilizing Activity	Usual Therapeutic Dose Range (mg/day)	Beta-Blocking Plasma Concentrations	Elimination Half-Life (hr)	Lipid Solubility	Urinary Recovery of Unchanged Drug (% of dose)
Acebutolol	+	+	+	400–800	0.2–2 μg/ml	about 8	—	—
Alprenolol	0	++	+	200–800	50–100 ng/ml	2–3	Strong	<1
Atenolol	+	0	0	100–400	0.2–0.5 μg/ml	6–9	—	40
Metoprolol	+	0	±	100–800	50–100 ng/ml	3–4	Weak	3
Oxprenolol	0	++	+	40–360	80–100 ng/ml	2	Weak	—
Pindolol	0	+++	+	2.5–30	50–150 ng/ml	3–4	Weak	40
Practolol	+	++	0	25–800	1.5–5 μg/ml	6–8	Weak	>90
Propranolol	0	0	++	80–480	50–100 ng/ml	3.5–6	Strong	<1
Sotalol	0	0	0	80–480	0.5–4 μg/ml	5–13	—	60
Timolol	0	±	0	5–40	25–10 ng/ml	4–5	—	20

scious with peripheral cyanosis, weak heart sounds, and an unmeasurable blood pressure. The ECG revealed sinus rhythm of 60 to 70 per minute with normal atrioventricular conduction, ST segments, and T waves. He was treated with metaraminol and glucagon following gastric lavage. Two hours after admission, the plasma level of the drug was 12,200 ng per ml. Complete recovery occurred within 12 hours without signs of cardiovascular depression.

2. A 17-year-old daughter of a hypertensive patient ingested over 10 gm of metoprolol combined with alcohol and diazepam.[16] Upon hospital admission 1 hour later she was found to be conscious but very drowsy. There was no cyanosis and respirations were not affected. Her blood pressure was 80/60 mm Hg and her radial pulse 72 per minute and regular. Heart sounds and pupillary reaction were normal. A resting electrocardiogram on admission showed no pathologic findings. She was admitted to the intensive care unit and had normal sinus rhythm throughout. Treatment consisted of fluids. Blood pressure rose slowly during the course of the first 3 hours to 90/80 mm Hg and later to the patient's normal level of 115/70 mm Hg. Pulse rate varied during monitoring between 80 and 85 per minute. Twelve hours after admission the patient was up and about in good condition. The concentration of metoprolol in plasma was 13,100 ng per ml measured 11 hours after ingestion. The patient made an uneventful recovery.

Oxprenolol. (noncardioselective, partial agonist activity, membrane depressant). Five cases of oxprenolol overdosage have been reported, with two fatalities:

1. A 29-year-old male committed suicide by ingesting over 300 mg of oxprenolol after drinking 11 pints of beer.[17]
2. A 57-year-old female ingested 112 40-mg tablets of oxprenolol (4480 mg). She was brought to the emergency department 20 minutes later in coma.[18] She was cold and clammy and had central cyanosis. Her pulse was not palpable and her blood pressure unrecordable. Heart sounds were soft with a ventricular rate of 36 per minute and she had bibasilar rales. The ECG revealed an idioventricular rhythm at a rate of 36. External cardiac massage and assisted respiration procedures were carried out. There was no response in pulse rate to intravenous atropine and isoproterenol. A transvenous pacing catheter could not capture the ventricle. The patient died in asystole 1 hour after arrival in the hospital. An autopsy revealed no gross structural abnormality of the circulatory system. The postmortem plasma drug level was approximately 400 ng per ml.
3. A 62-year-old male ingested a large amount of oxprenolol and diazepam.[19] He was brought to the hospital pulseless with cold, cyanotic extremities

TABLE 5–3. Summary of World Experience with β-Adrenoceptor Blocker Intoxication

Drug	Pt. No.	Age	Sex	Estimated Ingested Dose (mg)	Other drugs	Plasma level (ng/ml)	Heart rate (beats/min)
					Preantidote		
Alprenolol	1	32	F	12,800	0	1,300	
Atenolol	1	24	F	1,200	0		80
Metoprolol	1	19	M	10,000	0	12,200	60–72
	2	17	F	10,000	Alcohol, diazepam	13,100	72
Oxprenolol	2	57	F	4,480	0	400	36
	3	62	M	?	Diazepam	3,100	0
	4	39	F	3,000	0		Unobtainable
Pindolol	1	38	F	500	0	1,500	80
	2	24	F	250	Diazepam	660	110
Practolol	1	39	M	9,000	0	58,600	70
	2	39	F	5,000	0		100
Propranolol	1	45	M	2,000	0		80
	2	35	F		0	28,000	
	3	34	F	6,000	Alcohol	14,000	
	4	38	F		Codeine	16,000	
	5	22	M	4,000	0		50
	6	37	F	800	Diazepam, imipramine		50
	7	24	F	1,000	Alcohol		40→asystole
	8	41	M	5,100	?Alcohol		50→asystole
	9	65	M	800	0	1,536	50
	10	2	M	150	0		60
	11	3	F	150	0		120

Preantidote						
Blood Pressure (mm Hg)	Level of Consciousness	Convulsions	Blood Sugar	Congestive heart failure	Bronchospasm	ECG
60 systolic	Coma					
150/110	Alert	0		No	No	Normal
Not measurable	Alert	0		Yes	No	Normal
80/60	Drowsy	0			No	Normal
Not measurable	Coma	0		Yes	No	Idioventricular rhythm
Not measurable	Coma	0		No	Yes	Asystole, sinus bradycardia
Not measurable	Coma	Yes		No	No	Bradycardia-rate = 20
240/140	Alert	0		No	No	Normal
130/80	Coma	0	Normal	Yes	No	Sinus tachycardia, IVCD, (QRS.11/sec)
90/60	Alert	0		No	No	Normal
110/60	Alert	0		Yes	No	LBBB
120 systolic	Alert	0		No		Normal
110/70	Alert	0	Normal	?		Bradycardia-rate = 42, transient atrioventricular block
60 systolic		0		Yes		
Unobtainable	Coma	0		?	Yes	Asystole
Unobtainable	Coma	Yes		?		Bradycardia then asystole
Unobtainable	Coma	0		?		1st° AV block, RBBB
130 systolic	Coma	?	14 mg/dl	No		Sinus bradycardia, atrioventricular block
125/75	Drowsy	0	50 mg/dl	No		Normal

(continued)

TABLE 5–3.   (cont.)

Drug	Pt. No.	Age	Sex	Treatment	Result	Reference
Alprenolol	1	32	F	Supportive	Death	13
Atenolol	1	24	F	Supportive	Recovery	14
Metoprolol	1	19	M	Gastric lavage, furosemide, metaraminol, Glucagon	Recovery	15
	2	17	F	Supportive	Recovery	16
Oxprenolol	2	57	F	Unresponsive to atropine, isoproterenol, pacemaker	Death	18
	3	62	M	Unresponsive to atropine, epinephrine, responded to glucagon bronchospasm treated with terbutaline	Recovery	19
	4	39	F	Atropine, isoproterenol, epinephrine, pacemaker	Recovery	20
Pindolol	1	38	F	None	Recovery	22
	2	24	F	Fluids	Recovery	23
Practolol	1	39	M	Supportive	Recovery	24
	2	39	F	Supportive	Recovery	25
Propranolol	1	45	M	Supportive	Recovery	26
	2	35	F	None	Death	27
	3	34	F	None	Death	28
	4	38	F	None	Death	29
	5	22	M	Atropine, epinephrine	Recovery	30
	6	37	F	Unresponsive to isoproterenol, responded to glucagon	Recovery	31
	7	24	F	Unresponsive to atropine, responded to epinephrine	Recovery	32
	8	41	M	Epinephrine, isoproterenol, pacemaker	Recovery	7
	9	65	M	Isoproterenol	Recovery	33
	10	2	M	Glucose	Recovery	34
	11	3	F	Glucose	Recovery	34

after being supported by the ambulance crew. The admission ECG revealed asystole. After 35 minutes of resuscitative efforts which included intravenous isoproterenol and epinephrine infusions, a slow sinus rhythm of 32 was established. This increased to 68 beats per minute after 0.6 mg of intravenous atropine, and respirations also returned. Systolic blood pressure did not increase over 30 mm Hg. Further epinephrine by continuous infusion had no effect on heart rate or blood pressure over 1½ hours. Glucagon, 10 mg IV, produced an arterial blood pressure of 150 mm Hg within 60 seconds and an improvement in peripheral circulation. As the cardiovascular state improved, severe bronchospasm developed, which was treated successfully with IV terbutaline. A continuous infusion of glucagon 2 mg hourly was given over the next 5 hours, and improvement continued after its withdrawal. The patient was eventually discharged after an uncomplicated recovery. The oxprenolol plasma level was 3100 ng per ml.

4. A 39-year-old female ingested 3 gm of oxprenolol.[20] After arrival at the emergency unit she had a respiratory arrest and a mild generalized convulsion. The blood pressure was unrecordable and the pulse very feeble, but spontaneous respirations returned and the cardiac monitor showed sinus rhythm with a rate of 60 per minute. Two further brief convulsions occurred. Following transfer to the intensive care unit she had a cardiorespiratory arrest with the monitor showing a bradycardia of 20 per minute. She was artificially ventilated and external cardiac massage was maintained for 2 hours. She received atropine, epinephrine (intracardiac and intravenous), isoproterenol, and sodium bicarbonate. A pacemaker was inserted with 100 percent capture. After 2 hours, the blood pressure was obtained at 130/100 mm Hg and she reverted to a sinus rhythm of 80 per minute. Within 48 hours she was fully conscious and after 72 hours assisted ventilation was discontinued. She made a full recovery.

5. A 67-year-old male ingested 30 80-mg oxprenolol tablets (2400 mg) along with 25 thiazide-potassium (navidrex-K) tablets.[21] The major problem in his clinical presentation was hyperkalemia. The oxprenolol may have delayed the normal excretion of potassium by lowering cardiac output and blood pressure. The patient made an uneventful recovery following supportive measures.

Pindolol. (noncardioselective, partial agonist activity, weak membrane depressant). Two uncomplicated cases of pindolol self-poisoning have been reported:

1. A 38-year-old female ingested 500 mg of pindolol in a suicide attempt.[22] She had been receiving 30 to 40 mg of pindolol for treatment of hypertension. She presented 5 hours after the massive ingestion with a blood

pressure of 240/140 and a pulse rate of 80. Her electrocardiogram was normal and she remained alert and cooperative. Her plasma pindolol level was 1500 ng per ml. There were no further complications.

2. A 24-year-old female ingested 250 mg of pindolol along with 150 mg of diazepam.[23] She presented the following morning in coma with a blood pressure of 80 mm Hg and a pulse of 110 beats per minute. After infusion of fluids her blood pressure came up to 130 mm Hg. The electrocardiogram revealed a sinus rhythm of 110 with a QRS duration of 0.11 seconds. The blood sugar was normal and pulmonary congestion was noted on the chest roentgenogram. Twenty hours later the QRS duration on the electrocardiogram was 0.06 seconds and the chest roentgenogram was normal. The plasma pindolol level was 660 ng per ml and the patient made an uneventful recovery.

Practolol. (cardioselective, partial agonist activity, no membrane effect). Two nonfatal cases of practolol self-poisoning have been reported:

1. A 39-year-old male with mitral valve disease ingested 9 gm of practolol.[24] He had been taking 400 mg daily for arrhythmias. Three hours after the massive ingestion, he was taken to the hospital where his heart rate was 70 beats per minute and the blood pressure 90/70 mm Hg. There were no changes in his level of consciousness and no signs of cardiac decompensation. Over the next 2 hours his blood pressure rose to its usual level. The plasma level was 58.6 μg per ml. The patient's course was uncomplicated.
2. A 39-year-old female with mitral stenosis ingested 5000 mg of practolol and presented with signs of mild congestive heart failure.[25] Her blood pressure was 110/60 and the heart rate 100. There was intermittent blockage of the left bundle branch. She made an uneventful recovery with resolution of the conduction defect.

Propranolol. (noncardioselective, membrane depressant, no partial agonist effect). In addition to our four cases of propranolol intoxication, 11 other well-documented cases have been reported, with 3 fatalities. The large experience with propranolol intoxication reflects its wide use in clinical practice.

1. Wermut and Wojcicki[26] reported a case of a 45-year-old man who ingested 2000 mg of propranolol in a suicide attempt. He arrived at the hospital 2 hours later in good condition. Plasma levels were not measured. His heart rate was 80 beats per minute, with a normal pulse contour, and his systolic blood pressure was 120 mm Hg. The electrocardiogram showed normal sinus rhythm and his course was uncomplicated.

2. A 35-year-old female with a past history of psychiatric illness was found dead in her living room chair.[27] Toxicologic studies revealed a propranolol plasma level of 28,000 ng per ml, and 600 mg of ingested drug remained in her stomach. An exact cardiovascular cause for her death was not determined.

3. A 34-year-old female was found dead in bed having allegedly swallowed 6 gm of propranolol with a large amount of alcohol.[28] The plasma propranolol level was 14,000 ng per ml and there was a massive concentration of drug in the brain. An exact anatomic cause for death was not determined.

4. A 38-year-old female with schizophrenia was found dead in bed having ingested an unknown amount of propranolol and codeine.[29] The plasma level of propranolol was 16,000 ng per ml. An autopsy revealed no significant gross pathologic findings.

5. A 22-year-old male ingested 4 gm of propranolol in a suicide attempt.[30] The blood pressure was 110/70 mm Hg. Sinus bradycardia ranged from 50 to 42 per minute and did not change with injections of epinephrine. The heart rate increased somewhat after atropine. There was no evidence of impaired atrioventricular conduction. Hypoglycemia was not observed and the outcome was favorable.

6. A 37-year-old female attempted suicide with a mixed overdose of imipramine, and 800 mg of propranolol.[31] She presented in the emergency room cyanotic, cold, with marked distention of the neck veins. The pulse rate was 50 per minute and regular and the systolic blood pressure was 60 mm Hg. She was unresponsive to an isoproterenol infusion but responded dramatically to 10 mg of glucagon intravenously. The blood pressure rose to 95 mm Hg and the pulse rate to 70 beats per minute. Marked improvement was also observed in peripheral perfusion and the degree of neck vein distention. She had an uncomplicated recovery.

7. A 24-year-old female ingested 1000 mg of propranolol with beer and whiskey.[32] Two hours later she was admitted to the hospital with a pulse rate of 35 to 40 per minute and no blood pressure. Rhonchi were heard over the lung fields. Atropine was given intravenously but asystole developed. Cardiorespiratory resuscitative efforts were begun and the patient responded to intracardiac epinephrine. The patient's course thereafter was uncomplicated. Plasma drug levels were not measured.

8. A 41-year-old male with a history of chronic alcoholism ingested 5.1 gm of propranolol.[7] He arrived in the emergency room 2 hours later and was found to be comatose and cyanotic with a pulse rate of 50 beats per minute. The blood pressure was unobtainable and he experienced intermittent generalized convulsions. ECG showed a bradycardia without identifiable P waves. He developed asystole and required intensive supportive efforts and therapy which included 115 mg of isoproterenol

over 2½ days, a transvenous pacemaker, and intravenous epinephrine. He remained in a coma for 18 hours and eventually made an uneventful recovery after 65 hours on an isoproterenol drip infusion. Plasma levels were not measured.

9. A 65-year-old male ingested 800 mg of propranolol.[33] Two hours later he presented in coma with respiratory compromise. The blood pressure was unobtainable and the pulse rate was 50 beats per minute. The ECG demonstrated first degree heart block and right bundle branch block. He responded to intravenous isoproterenol with a normalization of blood pressure, ECG, and heart rate. Plasma renin activity was severely depressed during the acute intoxication and rose briskly as the drug effect wore off. Plasma propranolol level was 1536 ng per ml. The patient's ultimate course was unremarkable.

10, 11. Propranolol-induced hypoglycemia was seen in two healthy siblings, a boy aged 20 months and a 3-year-old girl, who ingested 150 mg between them.[34] The boy presented in stupor, with a systolic blood pressure of 130 mm Hg and a pulse rate of 60 beats per minute. The ECG showed sinus rhythm and periodic second degree atrioventricular block. The plasma glucose was 14 mg per 100 ml. He responded to intravenous glucose with a dramatic improvement in his level of consciousness. The electrocardiogram reverted to normal after 3 days. The girl presented with drowsiness and diaphoresis. Her blood glucose was 50 mg per dl. The ECG, pulse rate, and blood pressure were normal. She rapidly recovered after milk and sugar perorally. Ten days after admission an oral glucose tolerance test was performed in both children which was within normal limits.

Sotalol. (no cardioselectivity, no partial agonist effect, no membrane depressant action), and **Timolol** (weak partial agonist activity). There have been no reported cases of serious overdosage with these two agents.

DISCUSSION

Self-poisoning with β-adrenoceptor blocking drugs is uncommon, but is being reported with increasing frequency as the therapeutic indications for these agents continue to grow.[6] The main clinical features of massive overdosage include bradycardia, hypotension, low cardiac output, cardiac failure, and cardiogenic shock.[6,35] Bronchospasm may also occur, and respiratory depression can develop perhaps as a result of severe circulatory impairment or from a central drug effect. In severe intoxications, the myocardium may become relatively refractory to pharmacologic and electrical stimulation, and death occurs in asystole.[6]

Pharmacology. When properly administered, the β-adrenoceptor blocking drugs are relatively safe, with a wide margin between therapeutic and toxic dose levels.[35] Patients vary in their sensitivity to these drugs, however. Some patients have tolerated therapeutic doses of up to 4 gm of propranolol daily[10] and deliberate overdosage of both practolol[24,25] and propranolol[26] without serious adverse effects. Conversely, circulatory collapse may occur in patients with preexisting cardiac failure when sympathetic drive is inhibited by even a small dose of a β-adrenoceptor antagonist.

Variations in the pharmacologic properties of the different β-adrenoceptor blocking agents (partial agonist activity, cardioselectivity, membrane depressant action, lipid solubility) affect their therapeutic actions and adverse effects.[2-5] These individual differences may influence the clinical features in serious overdosage. In the therapeutic dose range, these drugs act primarily as antiadrenergic agents. In high dosages, some of the compounds (acebutolol, alprenolol, oxprenolol, propranolol) have membrane stabilizing or "quinidine"-like properties in addition to their β-adrenoceptor blocking effects.[4] Initially this property was thought to explain the antiarrhythmic potency of β-blockers; however, it is not an important action with usual doses.[4,8]

Some β-adrenoceptor blocking compounds have partial agonist or intrinsic sympathomimetic properties (acebutolol, alprenolol, oxprenolol, pindolol and practolol).[4] These agents cause a small agonist effect indicating that they stimulate as well as block the receptor. This action is dose-related, increasing in importance with larger plasma concentrations of drug.[4]

Some compounds are cardioselective (acebutolol, atenolol, metoprolol, practolol), that is, they antagonize β-receptors in the heart at lower doses than are required for other tissues.[4] This property is also dose-related, becoming less important with increasing plasma concentrations of drug.[4]

β-Adrenoceptor blocking drugs also vary in lipid solubility, metabolic and excretory pathways, and protein binding.[4]

Acute Toxicity in Man. β-Blocking compounds are all rapidly absorbed from the gastrointestinal tract.[4] The first critical signs of overdosage can appear 20 minutes after ingestion, but are more commonly seen within 1 to 2 hours.[35] The half-life of these compounds is usually short, ranging from 20 to 12 hours (Table 5-2).[4] A depressed cardiac output, however, which reduces both liver and kidney perfusion, can significantly increase the plasma half-life.[33] This might explain the prolonged therapeutic efforts (greater than 72 hours) required in some patients with massive overdosage where cardiac function is compromised. In most reported instances of oxprenolol and propranolol self-poisoning, there was a marked slowing in sinus heart rate with hypotension and circulatory collapse. In contrast, the two cases of intoxication with pindolol (partial agonist activity) were associated with hypertension and tachycardia. Interestingly intoxications with cardioselective agents (atenolol, metoprolol, and practolol) were not associated with profound bradycardia. Overt pulmonary edema was a rare occurrence in β-adrenoceptor self-poisoning unless the patient had underlying heart disease.[6,35]

The usual electrocardiographic manifestations of β-adrenoceptor blockade include first degree atrioventricular heart block (prolonged PR interval) and sinus bradycardia. With massive intoxications, disappearance of P waves, asystole, and intraventricular conduction defects may be seen.[35] An intraventricular conduction defect was seen in 3 of 4 patients treated for propranolol intoxication at our institution. The presence of the intraventricular conduction correlated temporally with the presence of high concentrations of propranolol in the plasma. The electrocardiogram normalized as the plasma level fell into the therapeutic range. The widening of the QRS complex may be related to the membrane depressant or "quinidine" effect of propranolol which can manifest itself with high doses of the drug.[4] An intraventricular conduction defect has been seen in self-poisoning with other β-blocking agents having membrane depressant activity[5,9] and is rarely described in massive intoxications with agents lacking this property.[35]

Bronchospasm is a well-known adverse effect in patients treated with β-adrenoceptor blocking drugs, and is more frequent with noncardioselective agents.[3,5] It is a rare complication of β-blocker therapy, or overdosage, except in patients who already have bronchospastic disease.[35] Respiratory arrest has also been described with β-blocker intoxication, especially with propranolol, and has been felt to be secondary to a central drug effect.[6,35]

Propranolol interferes with the glycogen-mobilizing effects of catecholamines.[3,5] Hypoglycemia has been described in patients treated with both insulin and propranolol.[5] Hypoglycemia has not been a prominent feature of β-blocker self-poisoning alone, however.[35] There has only been one report of hypoglycemia in two nondiabetic children who ingested 150 mg of propranolol.[34]

Changes in mental and neurologic status have been reported in patients treated with propranolol.[36,37] The drug is extremely lipid-soluble and readily crosses the blood-brain barrier to concentrate in brain tissue.[4] Changes in neurologic and mental status are less of a problem in drugs which are not as lipid-soluble.[3] Loss of consciousness has been described as a consequence of low cardiac output in patients treated with β-adrenoceptor blocking agents. However, changes in mental status and even coma have been seen without evidence of cardiovascular compromise in patients with propranolol self-poisoning. Convulsions have also been seen in patients with β-adrenoceptor blocker overdosage. The seizure activity has been a feature of self-poisoning with agents having both high lipophilicity and membrane depressant activity. Seizures are not a feature of β-blocker overdosage with agents lacking this membrane depressant effect. The convulsions seen with propranolol may be caused by a mechanism similar to that seen with intravenous lidocaine, a local anesthetic drug with membrane depressant properties.[9]

Plasma Drug Levels. β-Adrenoceptor intoxication may be difficult to recognize, especially when the drug is taken in combination with other drugs. Although plasma drug levels are available, they do not always reflect the degree of β-adrenoceptor blocker intoxication. Patients have different degrees of sympathetic tone and different metabolic characteristics, so that a specific blood level may produce different clinical signs in each patient.[38] Moreover, certain compounds (alprenolol, propranolol) yield active metabolites which are not detected in the plasma assay.[4] It is also well known that the β-adrenoceptor blocking effect appears to last far longer than the short plasma half-life would suggest. It is, therefore, important that the physician recognize the clinical manifestations of β-adrenoceptor blocker intoxication and not rely on plasma drug levels. Estimating the plasma concentrations of β-blocking drugs may confirm the self-poisoning, but this is of limited value in the immediate management of patients.

THERAPY

In most cases of β-adrenoceptor blocker self-poisoning, medical treatment has been successful. The majority of reported fatalities occurred in patients who never received medical attention.

All β-adrenoceptor blocker intoxications can be treated in a similar fashion. The major goals of treatment are: (1) to quickly remove any ingested tablets; (2) to counteract life-threatening cardiovascular and pulmonary effects; (3) to treat central nervous system disturbances.

General Measures. Optimum management of these patients requires intensive supportive care with facilities for continuous cardiac monitoring and ventilatory support. Because the effects of β-blocking drugs on the body last longer than their chemical half-life in the plasma, intensive care may have to be continued for several days.[6] The clinical manifestations of intoxication may occur as early as 20 minutes after ingestion of drug but are usually seen 1 to 2 hours later.[35] Sudden rapid deterioration with cardiovascular collapse is common.[35]

Removal of Drug. Gastric lavage and emesis may allow the tablets to be identified. However, they are unlikely to be sufficient in preventing serious poisoning unless performed early, since β-blocking drugs are absorbed rapidly. If the ingestion is recent, emesis should be initiated unless the patient is comatose, convulsing, or has lost the gag reflex. When these contraindications are present, endotracheal intubation should be performed, followed by gastric lavage with a large-bore tube. Activated charcoal, 5 to 10 times the estimated ingested dose or 30 to 50 gm can be given orally or by lavage. Sodium or magnesium sulfate 250 mg per kg can be given orally as a cathartic.

Hemodialysis is unlikely to rid the body of propranolol since the drug is greater than 95 percent protein bound. This measure has not been tried in gross overdosage, however. It may be possible to dialyze β-blocking drugs which are more water soluble and less protein bound than propranolol, but the value of this procedure has not been assessed.[6]

Bradycardia and Hypotension. Hypotension may be caused by bradycardia, depression of myocardial contractility, or a central nervous system effect.[8]

Patients should be monitored carefully for atrioventricular conduction defects and bradycardia. Should these occur, atropine, at 0.5 to 3.0 mg intravenously in adults[39] or 50 μg per kg intravenously in children, should be given to reduce unopposed vagal activity. If this is unsuccessful, isoproterenol infusion, 4 μg per minute may be useful, although occasionally larger infusions have been requried to completely overcome β-adrenoceptor blockade. In one recent report a total of 115 mg of isoproterenol were infused over 65 hours.[7] The isoproterenol dose should be monitored according to the response of the pulse and blood pressure. Hypotension may be aggravated by the peripheral vasodilatory effects of isoproterenol, in which case treatment with dobutamine,[40] a cardioselective β-adrenoceptor agonist may be substituted. With severe hypotension, treatment with α-vasoconstrictors such as norepinephrine and dopamine may be necessary. Glucagon, which increases heart rate and improves atrioventricular conduction by nonadrenergic mechanisms (not influenced by β-adrenoceptor blockade), may be useful in patients unresponsive to isoproterenol.[41] Glucagon is administered as an initial intravenous bolus of 50 μg per kg infused over 1 minute, followed by an intravenous infusion of 1 to 5 mg per hour; it may be used in conjunction with isoproterenol or dobutamine. A temporary transvenous pacemaker should be inserted if heart block or severe bradycardia cannot be readily controlled by pharmacologic means.[35]

In addition to its electrophysiologic effects, glucagon activates adenyl cyclase and enhances myocardial contractility by mechanisms different from catecholamines; its inotropic effect is not blocked by β-blockers.[19,31,41,42] It is felt to be the initial drug of choice for myocardial depression and hypotension in β-blocker self-poisoning,[31,42] although both epinephrine and norepinephrine have been proven efficacious.

Pulmonary. The physician should rapidly establish effective respiratory function in patients, creating an artificial airway if necessary. An adequate tidal volume should be maintained. Severe bronchoconstriction, although rare in self-poisoning may require isoproterenol inhalation in larger than usual doses. Aminophylline can be given as an initial 5.6 mg per kg intravenous bolus over 15 to 20 minutes, followed by a continuous infusion of 0.9 mg per kg per hour. Serum aminophylline levels should be maintained at 10 to 20 μg per ml. A β_2-adrenoceptor-stimulating drug can also be administered (e.g., terbutaline).

Hypoglycemia. Hypoglycemia is a rare complication of β-adrenoceptor blocker self-poisoning. This complication, if present, can be treated with glucose and/or glucagon.

Seizures. Seizure activity can be seen in β-adrenoceptor blocker overdosage secondary to hypotension, hypoxia, or hypoglycemia, and all these conditions should be corrected. Some β-blockers have central nervous system depressant actions and may also cause seizures.[43] Intravenous Valium has proven effective in controlling seizure activity in several patients.

β-Blocker Withdrawal. Most patients who are successfully treated for self-poisoning will have no late sequelae. Certain patients following treatment of intoxication, however, may become prone to β-adrenoceptor "withdrawal" effects[44] (aggravation of chest pain or myocardial infarction in patients with angina pectoris), and should be closely observed for this complication.

REFERENCES

1. Morrelli HF: Propranolol. Ann Intern Med 78: 913, 1973
2. Frishman W, Silverman R: Clinical Pharmacology of the new beta adrenergic blocking drugs. Part 3: Comparative clinical experience and new therapeutic applications. Am Heart J 98: 114, 1979
3. Frishman E, Silverman R, Strom J, et al.: Clinical pharmacology of the new beta adrenergic blocking drugs. Part 4: Adverse effects. Choosing a β-adrenoceptor blocker. Am Heart J 98: 256, 1979
4. Frishman, W: Clinical Pharmacology of the new beta adrenergic blocking drugs. Part 1. Pharmacodynamic and pharmacokinetic properties. Am Heart J 97: 663, 1979
5. Frishman W, Silverman R: Clinical pharmacology of the new beta adrenergic blocking drugs. Part 2. Physiologic and metabolic effects. Am Heart J 97: 797, 1979
6. Editorial: Self-poisoning with beta-blockers. Br Med J 1: 1010, 1978
7. Lagerfelt J, Matell G: Attempted suicide with 5.1G of propranolol. A case report. Acta Med Scand 199: 517, 1976
8. Nies AS, Shand D: Clinical pharmacology of propranolol. Circulation 52: 6, 1975
9. Nies AS: Pathophysiologic and pharmacological considerations in drug administra-

tion (cardiovascular disorders). In Melmon K, Morrelli H (eds): Clinical Pharmacology. New York: Macmillan, 1978, p 242

10. Boakes AJ, Boerre BH: Suicidal attempts with beta-adrenoceptor blocking agents. Br Med J 4: 675, 1973
11. Waal-Manning J: Hypertension: which beta-blocker? Drugs 12: 412–441, 1976
12. Johnsson G, Regardh CG: Clinical pharmacokinetics of β-adrenoceptors blocking drugs. Clin Pharmacokin 1: 233–263, 1976
13. Simonsen J, Worm K: Acute fatal alprenolol poisoning. Ugeskr. Laeger. 139: 2817–2818, 1977
14. Shanahan FL, Counihan TB: Atenolol self-poisoning (letter). Br Med J 2: 773, 1978
15. Moller BHJ: Letter: Massive intoxication with metoprolol. Br Med J 1: 222, 1976
16. Sire S: Metoprolol intoxication (letter). Lancet 2: 1137, 1976
17. Editorial: Death from an overdose of oxprenolol. Pharm J 208: 143, 1972
18. Khan A: Muscat-Baron JM: Fatal oxprenolol poisoning. Br Med J 1: 552, 1977
19. Ward DE, Jones B: Glucagon and beta-blocker toxicity. Br Med J 2: 151, 1976
20. Mattingly PC: Oxprenolol overdose with survival (letter). Br Med J 1: 776–777, 1977
21. Hume L, Forfar JC: Hyperkalemia and overdosage of antihypertensive agents (letter). Lancet 2: 1182, 1977
22. Thorpe P: Prindolol in hypertension. Med J Aust 58: 1242, 1971
23. Offenstadt G, Hericord P, Amstutz P: (letter): Voluntary poisoning with pindolol. Nouv Presse Med 5: 1539, 1976
24. Karhunen P, Hartel G: Suicidal attempt with practolol. Br Med J 2: 178–179, 1973
25. Verdera Cosmelli JT, Garcia Del Pozo JM, Lopez Morales J: Attempted suicide with practolol. Rev Esp Cardiol 29: 195–197, 1976
26. Wermut W, Wojcicki M: Suicidal attempt with propranolol. Br Med J 3: 591, 1973
27. Gault R, Monforte JR, Khasnabis S: A death involving propranolol (Inderal). Clin Toxicol 11: 295–299, 1977
28. Kristinsson J, Johannesson T: A case of fatal propranolol intoxication. Acta Pharmacol Toxicol (KBH) 41: 190, 1977
29. Turner JE, Cravey RH: A fatal case involving propranolol and codeine. Clin Toxicol 8: 271–275, 1975
30. Gdyra D, Billip-Tomecka A, Szajewsky JM: Case of poisoning with a 4-gram dose of propranolol. Pol Arch Med Wewn 50: 1341–1344, 1973
31. Kosinski EJ, Malindzak GS Jr: Glucagon and isoproterenol, in reversing propranolol toxicity. Arch Intern Med 132: 840–843, 1973
32. Frithz G: Toxic effects of propranolol on the heart. Br Med J 1: 769–770, 1976
33. Ducret F, Zech P, Perrot D, Moskovtchenko, Traeger J: Deliberate self-overdose with propranolol. Change in serum levels. Nouv Presse Med 7: 27–28, 1978
34. Hesse B, Pedersen JT: Hypoglycemia after propranolol in children. Acta Med Scand 193: 551–552, 1973
35. Favarel-Garrigues JC, Gbikpi-Benissan G, Poisot D, Cardinaud JP, Gabinski C: Toxicite Aiguë des beta-bloquants. Bordeau Med 11: 2623, 1978
36. Koehler K, Guth W: Schizophrenia-like psychosis following administration of propranolol. Munch Med Wochenschr 119: 443–444, 1977
37. Steinert J, Pugh CR: Two patients with schizophrenia-like psychosis after treatment with beta-adrenergic blockers. Br Med J 1: 790–791, 1979

38. Frishman W, Smithen C, Befler B, Kligfield P, Killip T: Non-invasive assessment of clinical response to oral propranolol. Am J Cardiol 35: 635, 1978
39. Richards DA, Prichard BN: Self-poisoning with beta-blockers. Br Med J 1: 1623, 1978
40. Sonnenblick EH, Frishman WH, LeJemtel TH: Dobutamine: a new synthetic cardioactive sympathetic amine. N Eng J Med 300: 17, 1979
41. Glick G, Parmley W, Wechsler AS, Sonnenblick EH: Glucagon. Circ Res 22: 789, 1968
42. Parmley WW: The role of glucagon in cardiac therapy. N Eng J Med 285: 801, 1971
43. Buiumsohn A, Eisenberg E, Jacob H, Frishman WH: Seizures and intraventricular conduction defect in propranolol poisoning. Ann Intern Med 91: 860–862, 1979
44. Frishman WH, Christodoulou J, Weksler B, et al.: Abrupt propranolol withdrawal in angina pectoris: effects on platelet aggregation and exercise tolerance. Am Heart J 95: 169, 1978

CHAPTER SIX

Beta-Adrenoceptor Blockade and Coronary Artery Surgery

William H. Frishman, Yasu Oka, Ronald M. Becker,
Joel Strom, Alan Kadish, Masayuki Matsumoto,
Louis Orkin, and Robert Frater

BETA-ADRENOCEPTOR blocking drugs are important therapeutic agents in the medical management of patients with angina pectoris, hypertension, cardiac arrhythmias, thyrotoxicosis, pheochromocytoma, and obstructive cardiomyopathies.[1] An increasing number of patients can be expected to present for surgical anesthesia while taking these drugs.

During the past several years, recommendations regarding treatment of patients receiving propranolol and scheduled for coronary artery bypass operations have varied widely. These recommendations have ranged from the complete withdrawal of therapy 2 weeks prior to surgery[2] to the continuation of therapy at the same or lesser dosage just prior to the operation.[3-6] There are reports associating the abrupt withdrawal of long-term propranolol therapy with an increase in angina, new arrhythmias, myocardial infarction, or sudden death.[7-9] These raise the issue as to whether the risk of such withdrawal before coronary bypass operation is greater than the risk of the purported myocardial depression attributed to interaction between residual β-adrenoceptor blockade and general anesthesia.

Recent retrospective and prospective reviews of consecutive coronary artery bypass operations, in which propranolol therapy was not withdrawn for medical indications, have failed to identify any deleterious interaction between anesthesia and preoperative propranolol administration.[3-6,10-17] Moreover, in animal studies, anesthetic agents commonly used for bypass operations have been shown not to potentiate the effects of propranolol.

In a previous study with patients who underwent coronary artery bypass surgery, our group found a higher incidence of postoperative arrhythmias and hypertension in individuals withdrawn from propranolol preoperatively, when compared to a population who either never received the drug, or had the drug maintained postoperatively.[18] We therefore undertook this prospective study to elucidate the mechanism for these phenomena. Our protocol was designed to seek answers to the following questions:

1. Are there hazards associated with either preoperative maintenance or withdrawal of propranolol therapy?
2. Are there hazards related to persisting β-blockade during intubation, general anesthesia and coronary artery bypass surgery?
3. Does persisting β-blockade lead to poor postoperative cardiac performance?
4. Does propranolol withdrawal contribute to the high incidence of hypertension and arrhythmias seen following coronary artery bypass surgery? If so, what are the mechanisms?
5. How should propranolol and other β-adrenoceptor blocking drugs be utilized in the perioperative periods?

PATIENTS AND METHODS

Fifty-four consecutive patients with stable angina pectoris, scheduled for elective coronary artery bypass and receiving long-term propranolol therapy, were entered in a randomized trial. They were compared with 17 patients scheduled for bypass operations and receiving no propranolol therapy prior to surgery (Group I). The 54 propranolol treated were randomized into three treatment groups (Table 6-1); 17 patients had propranolol therapy abruptly withdrawn 48 hours before the operation (Group II); 18 patients had therapy abruptly withdrawn 10 hours prior to surgery (Group III); 19 patients had their full propranolol dose until the morning of surgery, half the usual dose 2 hours prior to surgery and postoperatively, 1 mg intravenously every 4 hours for 36 to 48 hours (Group IV).

The population characteristics of the patient groups are noted in Table 6-2. The groups had similar resting hemodynamic function and preoperative coronary anatomy. There were no patients with ejection fractions below

TABLE 6-1.   Propranolol Treatment Groups in Patients Undergoing Coronary Artery Bypass Surgery

Group	Preoperative Therapy	Postoperative Therapy
I	None	None
II	Drug stopped 48 hours prior to surgery	None
III	Drug stopped 10 hours prior to surgery	None
IV	Full dose until morning of surgery: one-half dose 2 hours prior to surgery	1 mg IV every 4 hours

TABLE 6-2. Characteristics of Patient Groups

	Group I	Group II	Group III	Group IV
Patient number	17	17	18	19
Age (yrs)	59 ±1	53 ±2	55 ±2	56 ±2
Sex				
Male	11	11	12	11
Female	6	6	6	8
LVEDP (mm Hg)*	14 ±1	14 ±1	15 ±2	15 ±1
Number of grafts	2.3 0.2	2.3 0.2	2.4 0.2	2.5 0.2
Propranolol dose (mg/day)	—	154 ±18	151 ±15	133 ±20
Previous myocardial infarct				
(% of group)	23	23	28	26
Previous hypertension				
(% of group)	35	41	28	32

*Obtained just prior to induction of anesthesia.

0.45, ventricular aneurysms, preexisting arrhythmias, or coexisting valvular disease. Patients with resting heart rates of 55 beats per minute while on propranolol were excluded from randomization.

All patients received the same preanesthetic and anesthetic management. Premedication consisted of morphine sulfate 0.15 mg per kg and scopolamine 0.015 mg per kg, given intramuscularly 40 to 60 minutes before induction of anesthesia.

Following the intravenous administration of 3 mg D-tubocurarine or 1 mg pancuronium, patients were induced with thiopental (3 to 4 mg per kg) and 0.5 to 2 percent halothane in oxygen. After administration of succinylcholine (1.5 mg per kg) and topical anesthetic of the larynx (lidocaine 4 percent), the trachea was intubated with an appropriate size endotracheal tube. Anesthesia was maintained with halothane 0.5 to 1 percent supplemented with nondepolarizing muscle relaxants.

The coronary artery bypass was performed using standard techniques. The operative procedure was accomplished with the aid of cardiopulmonary bypass, hemodilution perfusion, and moderate total body hypothermia (28 to 32C). A single period of aortic cross-clamping was used for all distal anastomoses, with hypothermic hyperkalemic cardioplegia to protect the myocardium. Average time for each distal coronary anastomosis was 13 minutes. All patient ECGs were monitored continuously for approximately 3 days in a surgical intensive care unit.

Preoperative blood pressure and heart rate measurements were obtained 24 hours prior to surgery and in the operating room. Intravenous and intra-arterial cannulas were inserted under local anesthesia. Continuous tracings of blood pressure and lead II (ECG) were recorded. Before induction of anesthesia, the presence of angina pectoris or arrhythmias was noted. During the course of anesthesia and postoperatively, hemodynamic measures included blood pressure, heart rate, arrhythmias, and the displacement of the ECG ST-segment. The heart rate-blood pressure product (RPP), and indirect measure of myocardial oxygen consumption, was also calculated.[19-20]

For purposes of tabulation, hemodynamic observations were summarized according to the following time periods: (1) 24 hours prior to surgery; (2) in operating room prior to anesthesia induction; (3) intubation; (4) 1 hour of anesthesia; (5) 15 minutes postoperatively (intensive care unit); (6) 1 to 2 hours postoperatively; (7) 24 hours postoperatively. Also noted were the rate of recovery of cardiac function following cardiopulmonary bypass and the need for cardiotonic drugs. Postoperative complications as well as the need for cardioactive agents until hospital discharge were recorded.

To establish plasma propranolol levels, blood specimens were obtained at the time of induction, after cardiopulmonary bypass and immediately upon arrival in the intensive care unit. Measurements were made using the modified fluorometric method of Coltart and Shand.[21] Blood specimens for plasma renin activity were obtained several times: in the operating room prior to induction (control); 5 minutes after intubation; and, following surgery (15 minutes, and 2 hours). The renin measurements were made by the radioimmunoassay technique of Chervu et al.[22]

The significance of differences between groups was determined by chi square analysis and that of differences in means by Student's t test for nonpaired data. The standard error of the mean was used as the index of dispersion.

RESULTS

The four patient groups were remarkably homogenous for mean characteristics such as sex, history of hypertension and previous myocardial infarction, duration of anesthesia, duration of cardiopulmonary bypass, and number of coronary vessels bypassed. There were no differences between the groups in the ease of discontinuing cardiopulmonary bypass.

There were five perioperative infarctions (new Q waves) seen and one death. The incidence of infarction among the different groups was Group I, 6 percent (1 out of 17); Group II, 18 percent (3 out of 17); Group III, 6 percent (1 out of 18); Group IV, 0 percent (none out of 19). The one death occurred in a Group II patient, 28 hours after surgery, from low cardiac output as a consequence of infarction.

Hemodynamic results are shown in Figures 6-1 to 6-6 and Table 6-3. During the control period (24 hours prior to surgery), patients in Groups III and IV (both still receiving propranolol) had significantly lower mean RPP than did Group I and II patients. Immediately prior to surgery patients in Groups III and IV continued their significantly lower RPP.

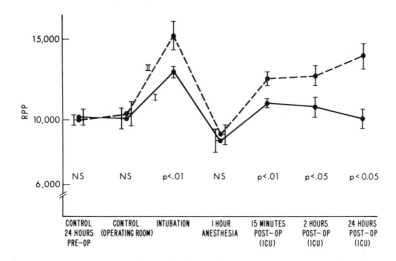

Figure 6-1.   Mean RPP of Group I patients (no propranolol) and Group II patients (propranolol discontinued 48 hours preoperatively) before, during, and after coronary artery surgery. Group I is shown with a solid line. Group II is shown with a broken line. Group II patients demonstrate a significant increment in RPP during intubation and the postoperative intervals when compared to Group I patients. The P values refer to the differences between groups at the different study intervals. NS = not significant.

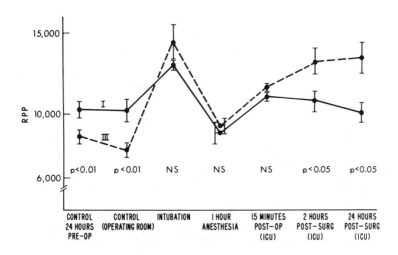

Figure 6-2.   Mean RPP of Group I patients (no propranolol) and group III patients (propranolol discontinued 10 hours preoperatively) before, during and after coronary artery surgery. Group I is shown with a solid line; Group III with a broken line. Group III patients had significantly lower RPP (probably due to persistence of β-adrenoceptor blocker effect) than group I during the preoperative intervals. With intubation there is no difference between groups, however. Two hours and 24 hours postoperatively, the RPP is signficantly higher in Group III patients compared to Group I.

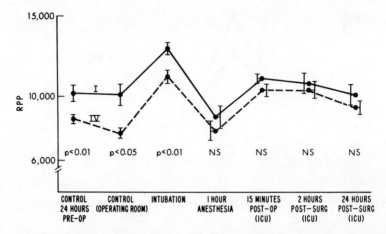

Figure 6-3. Mean RPP of Group I patients (no propranolol) and Group IV patients (propranolol maintained until 2 hours preoperatively, restarted immediately postoperatively) before, during, and after coronary artery surgery. Group I is shown with a solid line; Group IV with a broken line. Group IV patients had significantly lower RPP than Group I patients during the preoperative intervals. The increment in RPP with intubation was significantly blunted in Group IV patients. The operative and postoperative differences in RPP between groups were not signficantly different.

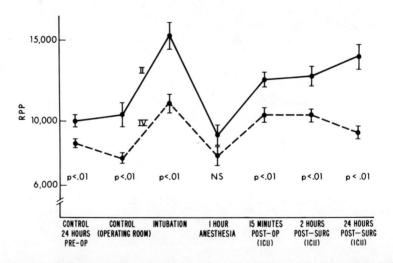

Figure 6-4. Mean RPP of Group II patients (propranolol discontinued 48 hours preoperative) and Group IV patients (propranolol maintained until 2 hours preoperatively, restarted immediately) before, during, and after coronary artery surgery. Group II is shown with a solid line; Group IV with a broken line. Group IV patients had significantly lower RPP at each study interval compared to Group II patients.

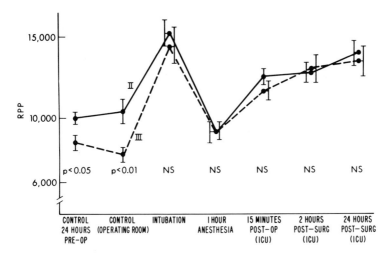

Figure 6-5. Mean RPP of Group II patients (propranolol discontinued 48 hours preoperatively) and Group III patients (propranolol discontinued 10 hours preoperatively) before, during, and after coronary artery surgery. Group II is shown with a solid line; Group III with a broken line. Group III patients had significantly lower RPP during the preoperative periods, however, there were no differences between the groups during the other study intervals. A marked increment in RPP during intubation and the postoperative periods was seen.

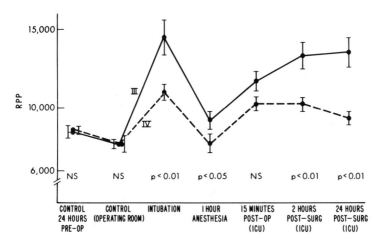

Figure 6-6. Mean RPP of Group III patients (propranolol discontinued 10 hours preoperatively) and Group IV patients (propranolol maintained until 2 hours preoperatively, restarted immediately postoperatively) before, during, and after coronary artery surgery. Group III is shown with a solid line; Group IV with a broken line. There were no differences between the groups during the preoperative control periods. However, there were significant increments in RPP during intubation and the postoperative periods in Group III patients compared to Group IV patients.

103

TABLE 6-3.   Effects of Different Propranolol Regimens on Heart Rate, Systolic Blood Pressure, and Rate Pressure Product in Patients Undergoing Coronary Artery Bypass Surgery

Observation Period	Group I	Group II	Group III	Group IV
Control (24 hr preop)				
Heart rate	79 ± 3	76 ± 3	72 ± 2	70 ± 2
Blood pressure	131 ± 4	132 ± 3	122 ± 6	125 ± 3
Rate pressure product	10,200 ± 485	10,000 ± 364	8,500 ± 436	8,600 ± 252
Control (immediate preop)				
Heart rate	78 ± 4	79 ± 3	66 ± 5	67 ± 3
Blood pressure	130 ± 6	132 ± 4	118 ± 5	114 ± 3
Rate pressure product	10,100 ± 655	10,400 ± 752	7,700 ± 485	7,700 ± 275
Intubation				
Heart rate	71 ± 2	80 ± 2	84 ± 4	71 ± 3
Blood pressure	180 ± 7	190 ± 6	173 ± 7	154 ± 5
Rate pressure product	13,000 ± 364	15,300 ± 846	14,500 ± 1,116	11,200 ± 458
1 hr anesthesia				
Heart rate	73 ± 4	76 ± 4	75 ± 3	66 ± 1
Blood pressure	115 ± 5	120 ± 4	125 ± 7	108 ± 4
Rate pressure product	8,742 ± 723	9,100 ± 631	9,235 ± 543	7,817 ± 596
15 min postop (ICU)				
Heart rate	84 ± 3	97 ± 3	88 ± 2	80 ± 3
Blood pressure	132 ± 3	131 ± 4	132 ± 5	135 ± 4
Rate pressure product	11,100 ± 242	12,600 ± 436	11,700 ± 631	10,400 ± 435
2 hrs postop (ICU)				
Heart rate	84 ± 7	96 ± 4	92 ± 5	79 ± 2
Blood pressure	130 ± 4	136 ± 3	144 ± 7	136 ± 3
Rate pressure product	10,800 ± 655	12,800 ± 582	13,300 ± 800	10,400 ± 435
24 hrs postop (ICU)				
Heart rate	84 ± 2	105 ± 5	96 ± 3	77 ± 2
Blood pressure	116 ± 3	137 ± 7	140 ± 7	120 ± 4
Rate pressure product	10,100 ± 582	14,000 ± 776	13,400 ± 946	9,300 ± 389

		Statistical Significance			
GROUP I VS GROUP II	GROUP I VS GROUP III	GROUP I VS GROUP IV	GROUP II VS GROUP III	GROUP II VS GROUP IV	GROUP III VS GROUP IV
NS	NS	<0.01	NS	NS	NS
NS	NS	NS	NS	NS	NS
NS	<0.01	<0.01	<0.05	<0.01	NS
NS	<0.01	<0.01	<0.05	<0.01	NS
NS	NS	<0.01	<0.05	<0.01	NS
NS	<0.05	<0.05	<0.01	<0.01	NS
<0.01	<0.01	NS	NS	<0.05	<0.05
NS	NS	<0.05	NS	<0.01	<0.01
<0.01	NS	<0.01	NS	<0.01	<0.01
NS	NS	<0.05	NS	<0.05	<0.05
NS	NS	NS	NS	<0.05	<0.05
NS	NS	NS	NS	NS	<0.05
<0.01	NS	NS	<0.05	<0.01	<0.05
NS	NS	NS	NS	NS	NS
<0.01	NS	NS	NS	<0.01	NS
NS	NS	NS	NS	<0.01	<0.05
NS	NS	NS	NS	NS	NS
$p<0.05$	$p<0.05$	NS	NS	<0.01	<0.01
<0.01	<0.01	<0.05	NS	<0.01	<0.01
<0.01	<0.01	NS	NS	<0.05	<0.05
<0.05	<0.05	NS	NS	<0.01	<0.01

Group I: No propranolol
Group II: Propranolol stopped 48 hours preoperatively.

Group III: Propranolol stopped 10 hours preoperatively.
Group IV: Propranolol stopped 2 hours preoperatively, continued postoperatively.

With intubation there was a dramatic increase in RPP in all four groups, predominantly due to a marked systolic blood pressure elevation (in some patients up to 280 mm Hg). However, the RPP increment in Group IV patients was significantly blunted compared to Groups I to III. This resulted in a RPP value for Group IV that was significantly lower than the other three groups. Group I patients (no propranolol) also had a lower RPP increment than Groups II and III.

After 1 hour of halothane anesthesia the blood pressure and RPP had returned to near control levels (24 hours preoperatively) for all groups; however, Group IV continued to have a significantly lower RPP than the other three groups.

Fifteen minutes following surgery, in the ICU, the RPP was found to rise in all four groups (though not as markedly as during intubation). Group II patients had the highest increment in both pulse rate and RPP compared with the three other groups.

Two hours later, patients in Group III were found to have a greater increment in heart rate and RPP compared to 15 minutes postoperatively. At this point, Groups II and III were similar with a higher heart rate and RPP than Groups I and IV.

Twenty-four hours postsurgery, the heart rate, blood pressure, and RPP continued to climb in both Groups II and III (with the RPP approaching the level found during intubation). Blood pressure, heart rate, and RPP in Groups I and IV remained significantly lower than in Groups II and III.

There was a significant difference in the incidence of supraventricular arrhythmias among the four study groups during the initial 24 hour postoperative period (Table 6-4, Figure 6-7). In Group I, 7 patients remained in normal sinus rhythm, and 10 developed supraventricular arrhythmias (6 sinus tachycardia >110, 4 paroxysmal supraventricular tachycardia or atrial flutter). Group II patients had the highest incidence of supraventricular arrhythmias among the four study groups. One patient remained in normal sinus rhythm, and sixteen developed supraventricular arrhythmias (8 sinus

TABLE 6-4.   Incidence of Postoperative (24 Hours) Supraventricular Tachyarrhythmia Following Coronary Artery Bypass

	Group I	Group II	Group III	Group IV
No. of patients	17	17	18	19
Normal sinus rhythm	7	1	3	14
Supraventricular tachyarrhythmias	10	16	15	5
Sinus tachycardia →110	6	8	7	3
Paroxysmal atrial tachyarrhythmias*	4	8	8	2

*Paroxysmal atrial tachycardia, atrial fibrillation, atrial flutter.

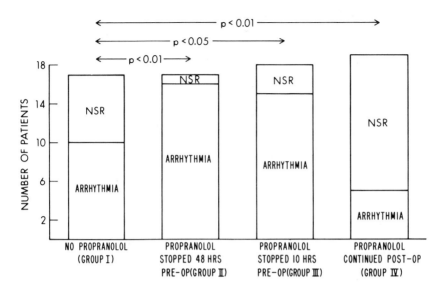

Figure 6-7.   The incidence of supraventricular arrhythmias postcoronary artery bypass in the different propranolol treatment groups. There was a significant increase in the frequency of arrhythmias in Group II patients (propranolol discontinued 48 hours preoperatively) and Group III patients (propranolol discontinued 10 hours preop) compared to Group I (no propranolol). Group IV patients (propranolol maintained postoperatively) had a significantly lower incidence of arrhythmias compared to Group I patients (no propranolol).

tachycardia >110, and 8 paroxysmal supraventricular tachycardia or atrial flutter-fibrillation). Group III patients also had a high incidence of supraventricular arrhythmias (7 sinus tachycardia >110, 8 paroxysmal supraventricular tachycardia or atrial flutter-fibrillation). In Group IV, 14 patients were in normal sinus rhythm and 5 developed arrhythmias (3 sinus tachycardia >110 and 2 paroxysmal atrial tachycardia or atrial flutter-fibrillation). The incidence of arrhythmia was significantly higher in Group II ($p < 0.01$) and Group II ($p < 0.05$) when compared to Groups I and IV. Group IV had a significantly lower incidence of supraventricular arrhythmia than the other three treatment groups ($p < 0.01$). All paroxysmal arrhythmia episodes, in each group, responded to intravenous propranolol (or supplementary propranolol in Group IV patients). Ventricular arrhythmias were rarely seen in the initial 24 hour postoperative period.

Plasma renin activity (PRA) was lower in Group IV patients, as compared to all other groups, throughout the control, intubation, and postoperative periods. There were no significant differences in PRA between Groups II, III, and IV during the intubation and postoperative intervals. Comparing Groups I and IV, the results were: Control (operating room) Group I, 1.13 ± 0.04 ng per ml per hour; Group IV, 0.96 ± 0.11 ng per ml per hour; after intubation Group I, 1.36 +0.26 ng per ml per hour; Group IV, 0.98 ±0.12 ng per ml per hour; 15 minutes postoperation Group I, 1.86 ± 0.10 ng per ml per hour; Group IV, 0.95 ±0.15 ng per ml per hour (p< 0.01); 2 hours postoperation Group I, 1.66 ±0.53 ng per ml per hour, Group IV, 1.08 +0.19 ng per ml per hour.

Propranolol plasma levels at the time of intubation were negligible for Group II patients, and 9.32 ±0.82 ng per ml per hour in Group III patients (minimal therapeutic level was 40 ng per ml). One hour after cardiopulmonary bypass, the drug level in Group III declined progressively to 3.75 ±0.30 ng per ml, so that in the immediate postoperative period it was negligible, 2.26 ±0.22 ng per ml. Renal clearance of propranolol increased considerably during cardiopulmonary bypass. Group IV patients had a plasma propranolol level of 39.1 ±1.17 ng per ml at the time of induction which decreased considerably postcardiopulmonary bypass to 5.2 ±0.80 ng per ml.

DISCUSSION

Although the therapeutic value of β-blockers is well established for angina pectoris, hypertension, arrhythmias, hypertrophic obstructive cardiomyopathy, thyrotoxic tachycardia, and pheochromocytoma,[1] the attitudes of anesthesiologists and surgeons concerning their use during anesthesia and surgery range from enthusiasm to frank antagonism. This debate has recently extended to the anesthetic management of patients who are undergoing coronary artery bypass surgery and receiving propranolol for the treatment of angina pectoris. Like the earlier controversy concerning antihypertensive therapy (with reserpine), evidence for withholding β-adrenoceptor blockade prior to elective anesthesia and surgery is sparce and largely anecdotal. Many cardiologists are properly reluctant to withdraw a form of therapy on which their patients are highly dependent, since the consequences of withdrawal may be increased angina pectoris, myocardial infarction, and death. Thus, those who recommend abrupt withdrawal of these drugs prior to elective coronary artery surgery should have compelling evidence that patients receiving β-blockers are at significantly more risk during anesthesia and surgery than if these agents are withdrawn. This study provides no such evidence. Rather, the data demonstrate that continuation of propranolol up to surgery, and its reinstitution postoperatively, protects angina pectoris patients from the undesirable sequelae of laryngoscopy, intubation, and the stresses of the postoperative period.

Theoretical potential dangers of anesthesia in patients taking β-blockers have been advanced since 1964.[24] The contention in these early reports was that β-adrenoceptor blockade would result in profound myocardial depression during general anesthesia.

Propranolol-induced myocardial depression has been implicated in the postoperative left ventricular failure occasionally seen after coronary artery surgery. In 1972, Viljoen et al.[2] described five patients with advanced coronary artery disease who received propranolol (100 to 320 mg) to within 24 hours of surgery: four died and one had a stormy postoperative course. The authors concluded that propranolol was a major factor in these deaths and recommended that it be discontinued for two weeks before operations. However, close scrutiny reveals that these five cases were complicated by other factors, and it is difficult to implicate propranolol as the sole cause of the complications seen. In 1973, Faulkner et al.[25] demonstrated that negative inotropic effects of propranolol had disappeared within 48 hours. They suggested that the recommendation of Viljoen for a two week preoperative withdrawal period was unfounded.

In 1974, Caralps and his associates[10] reviewed 100 cases of coronary artery bypass, including 25 patients receiving 40 to 200 mg of propranolol 24 hours or less before surgery. They found that the operative course of patients receiving propranolol, many of whom had unstable angina, was no different from that of untreated patients. In a larger review of 303 patients who underwent coronary artery surgery, the same investigators found that propranolol-treated subjects (48 hours or less prior to surgery) not only tolerated the operative procedure well, but also demonstrated lower mortality (3.8 percent for patients receiving propranolol versus 6.6 percent for those never receiving the drug).[11]

In 1975, Kaplan and his associates[17] reviewed the records of 169 patients undergoing coronary artery bypass, of whom 143 had been taking propranolol, with regard to preoperative administration of propranolol and intraoperative or postoperative complications. Patients taking propranolol until 24 hours before surgery showed no increased incidence of hypotension or bradycardia before cardiopulmonary bypass. Hypotension after bypass was no more common in patients off propranolol 12 to 48 hours than in patients who were discontinued more than 48 hours before operation or had never taken the drug. The operative mortality rate was 4 percent in patients taking propranolol within 48 hours of surgery and 6 percent in all other patients. The authors concluded that propranolol could be given safely within 12 to 48 hours of coronary artery surgery. Kaplan and Dunbar,[12] in 1976, also showed that patients with angina pectoris undergoing noncardiac surgical procedures and general anesthesia could safely tolerate propranolol administration to within 24 hours of operation.

The relative safety of maintaining propranolol just prior to surgery, established by these retrospective studies, emphasized the need for a prospective study to delineate the true clinical interaction between propranolol and general anesthesia for coronary artery operations.[9] Reports associating the abrupt withdrawal of long-term propranolol therapy with an increase in angina pectoris, new arrhythmias, myocardial infarction or sudden death, raised the issue as to whether the risk of such withdrawal before coronary bypass operation was greater than the risk of purported myocardial depression.[7-9]

The mechanism for the withdrawal reaction is unknown. Since propranolol lowers myocardial oxygen requirements, abrupt withdrawal of the drug may then raise the oxygen requirements beyond what the coronary arteries can supply, resulting in severe ischemia or myocardial infarction.[26,27] Other postulated mechanisms include increased platelet aggregability,[28] hypersensitivity to circulating catecholamines (analogous to denervation hypersensitivity),[29] and reactivation of the renin-angiotensin aldosterone mechanism.[27]

In a recent editorial, Shand and Wood[26] stated their belief that the propranolol withdrawal syndrome was real but rare. Shiroff and his associates[30] found the syndrome to be rare in patients with angina pectoris who had their propranolol stopped abruptly prior to cardiac catheterization. The effect may have been blunted in Shiroff's series because these patients had reduced in-hospital physical activity. A rebound effect following propranolol withdrawal may be more important in the setting of surgical stress, however. There is evidence that catecholamines and the level of adrenergic tone are elevated during laryngoscopy and intubation,[31-36] and again after saphenous vein coronary bypass.[16,37-48] There are marked increments in blood pressure demonstrated during intubation, and a marked increase in heart rate, blood pressure, and arrhythmias in the immediate postoperative state.[16,31-43] Patients who have their propranolol stopped abruptly may become hypersensitive to catecholamines during these periods.[29]

In a retrospective study by Langou et al.[49] the risk of perioperative myocardial infarction was significantly increased by abrupt propranolol withdrawal 24 hours before coronary surgery, as compared to a gradual withdrawal regimen (32 percent infarct rate versus 7.3 percent infarct rate). Recent studies by Kirsh et al.,[5] Kopriva et al.,[14] and Boudoulas et al.[16] demonstrated the safety of propranolol administered within 1 to 5 hours of coronary artery surgery.

In a large prospective trial by Slogoff et al.,[4] chronic propranolol therapy was administered in full dosage just prior to surgery and comparison made to patient groups where therapy was not given or abruptly withdrawn 24 to 72 hours preoperatively. Patients abruptly withdrawn from their propranolol treatment had the highest incidence of intraoperative ischemia and arrhythmias. This is probably related to a higher RPP than was seen in patients where propranolol was maintained just prior to surgery. Hypotension and bradycardia were not increased in patients who had propranolol continued. Moreover, no differences among groups were noted in ease of discontinuation of cardiopulmonary bypass, need for cardiac stimulants or in mortality.

In another recent prospective study, Boudoulas et al.[3] demonstrated that propranolol maintained prior to surgery lowered the incidence of su-praventricular tachyarrhythmias in the postoperative period, when com-pared to patients where propranolol was abruptly discontinued 24 hours prior to surgery. There were no complications related to propranolol during the intraoperative period. The left ventricular function, as measured from systolic time intervals, was the same pre- and postoperatively with both treatment regimens.

Patients with angina pectoris who had propranolol withdrawn more than 48 hours prior to surgery demonstrated a high incidence of supraven-tricular arrhythmias and hypertension, following coronary artery bypass, when compared to patients who had the drug maintained just prior to sur-gery.[18] We postulated a propranolol withdrawal effect as the cause for these phenomena. Therefore, we designed our study utilizing different preopera-tive propranolol treatment regimens to be compared with the control of no previous propranolol therapy.

Our results show that propranolol can be given safely to hemodynam-ically stable patients just before undergoing elective coronary artery bypass surgery. Propranolol-treated patients (Group IV — drug maintained just prior to surgery and resumed postoperatively) had a significant blunting of the hypertensive reflex usually seen during intubation,[31] and demonstrated negligible changes in the rate-pressure product in the postoperative period. A significant reduction in the incidence of supraventricular arrhythmias was also noted. Of concern was the finding that there were greater in-crements in systolic blood pressure and RPP during the intubation and postoperative periods, in those patients where propranolol was stopped 10 to 48 hours prior to surgery (Groups II, III), when compared to Group I (no propranolol), and Group IV patients. There was also a significantly higher incidence of arrhythmias seen in those patients who had propranolol abruptly withdrawn as compared to Group IV.

The data in this report suggest that there is a true propranolol "with-drawal effect" which becomes manifest during coronary artery surgery. This phenomenon does not appear to be mediated by the renin-angiotensin system, as was previously suggested,[50,51] but probably by a hyperadrenergic response to a stress situation.[16] The patients who never received propranolol did not demonstrate a large increment in rate-pressure product in the post-operative period, despite having higher serum renin activity when com-pared to Group IV patients (propranolol maintained). The marked incre-ments in rate-pressure product (an indirect index of myocardial oxygen de-mand)[19,20] and frequency of arrhythmia, in the postoperative periods, was a specific finding in those patients who had propranolol abruptly withdrawn. Patients who had propranolol maintained just prior to surgery (Group IV) failed to demonstrate this postoperative rate-pressure product of ar-rhythmia increment. Catecholamines were not measured, so it is not known whether the postoperative rate-pressure product increments in this study are secondary to increased catecholamine levels and/or adrenoceptor hypersensitivity, as is suggested by others.[16,29,39]

In this study, the finding that those patients who were withdrawn just 10 hours prior to surgery were not protected from marked increments in rate-pressure product during the operation (intubation) and postoperative period was surprising, in light of the alleged prolonged pharmacodynamic half-life of propranolol,[52,53] which contrasts to its shorter pharmacokinetic half-life.[54,55] This might be explained by the increased clearance of the drug during cardiopulmonary bypass and the heightened adrenergic state in the immediate postoperative period. Following cardiopulmonary bypass, negligible plasma drug levels were found in Groups III and IV, reinforcing a need to maintain propranolol intravenously during the immediate postoperative period to protect against the postoperative adrenergic state.[37-41]

There are important clinical implications of this study. First, increased myocardial oxygen demands during intubation may be even more important than a compromised blood supply in causing ischemia. Findings of intubation-induced hypertension and tachycardia have been demonstrated in many studies, emphasizing the need to protect patients (with β-adrenergic blockade) from this catecholamine mediated phenomenon.[31-36] Moreover, a propranolol withdrawal effect, following an abrupt premature discontinuation of the drug, may further aggravate this phenomenon.[29] Many of the perioperative myocardial infarctions observed with coronary bypass surgery[56] may relate to the intubation-related increase in rate-pressure product, an effect which usually persists for 5 minutes.[34] In this study, five myocardial infarctions were seen in Group II and Group III versus none in Group IV.

Second, there is probably no need to give propranolol during the operative period. Halothane and enflurane are the general anesthetics most commonly used for coronary artery bypass surgery and, like propranolol, are myocardial depressants (agents that will lower the oxygen demand of the heart).[57] The drugs have been shown to decrease the activity of the sympathetic nervous system and to reduce the output of catecholamines by adrenergic nerve endings and the adrenal medulla. Direct effects on autonomic nerve terminals have not been demonstrated and there is no reason to believe, nor any evidence to support, the notion that halothane may act on adrenal receptors.[57] As demonstrated in this report, patients in all four groups had similar low RPP after 1 hour of halothane anesthesia. The effects of propranolol and halothane are usually additive and not potentiated with the concentrations of halothane used in coronary artery surgery.[58]

Third, the well-documented hyperadrenergic state in the early postoperative period,[37-42] may explain the high incidence of hypertension and arrhythmias reported in this study.[37-41] Intravenous maintenance propranolol appears to blunt this stress reaction whereas premature propranolol withdrawal seems to aggravate it. The supraventricular arrhythmias appear to be catecholamine-mediated, since they all respond to intravenous propranolol therapy. Unlike propranolol the efficacy of digoxin in treating postoperative arrhythmias has not been demonstrated.[59]

Maintenance of myocardial oxygen demands at relatively low levels with propranolol might be especially important in the prebypass operative period in patients undergoing complete coronary artery revascularization. The demonstration that perioperative myocardial infarction often occurs in the period between anesthesia induction and onset of cardiopulmonary bypass emphasizes the need for myocardial protection during this most vulnerable period.[60,61] During the postbypass period, myocardial oxygen demands should also be controlled, especially in patients who undergo incomplete coronary revascularization procedures, where threatened myocardium may still remain, or in noncardiac operative procedures for patients with angina pectoris, where the entire myocardium may remain threatened.

The mortality of patients with angina pectoris undergoing elective noncardiac procedures has been reported to be three times higher than that of patients undergoing elective coronary revascularization procedures.[62] Proper anesthetic technique and careful hemodynamic monitoring are important for all patients with ischemic coronary artery disease who undergo cardiac or noncardiac operations. In this study, all the perioperative myocardial infarctions were seen in those patients who either had propranolol abruptly withdrawn or never received the drug preoperatively.

Many of the newer β-adrenoceptor blocking agents (i.e., practolol — cardioselective; pindolol — intrinsic sympathomimetic activity; alprenolol, labetalol — α- and β-blocking activity) have been evaluated during surgical procedures and, like propranolol, were found to be well tolerated.[33,63-68] Since all the β-adrenoceptor blocking agents have similar effects on angina pectoris, arrythmia and hypertension, the danger of abrupt treatment withdrawal with these agents should parallel that seen with propranolol.[69]

CONCLUSION

1. Propranolol can safely be maintained just prior to coronary artery surgery in hemodynamically stable patients and resumed in the immediate postoperative period with no difficulty.

2. Propranolol blunts the profound increases seen in myocardial oxygen demand during intubation and postoperative periods. These increments appear to be catecholamine-mediated and are unrelated to the renin-angiotensin system.

3. There is a demonstrable propranolol withdrawal effect when the drug is stopped abruptly 10 to 48 hours prior to coronary artery surgery. This appears to aggravate the hyperadrenergic state seen during the intubation and postoperative periods.

4. There is a rapid clearance of propranolol during cardiopulmonary bypass with disappearance of the drug, demonstrating the need to tempor-
   arily restart the drug in the immediate postoperative period where adrenergic tone is high.
5. There is a high incidence of supraventricular arrhythmias seen in patients where propranolol is withdrawn abruptly 10 to 48 hours prior to
   surgery. The arrhythmias are probably catecholamine-mediated since
   they are prevented by propranolol prophylaxis and respond readily to
   treatment with propranolol.
6. The recognition of a propranolol withdrawal effect during cardiac surgery raises an even greater concern for those patients with chronic angina pectoris who, receiving propranolol prior to undergoing noncardiac
   surgical procedures, are abruptly withdrawn.

RECOMMENDATIONS

We strongly believe that with the proper indications for its use, chronic
therapy with propranolol should be continued in moderate doses to the
time of surgery. (We recommend half the usual dose be given orally 2 hours
prior to surgery and restarting intravenous propranolol immediately postoperatively.) Not only will this minimize the occurrence of complications of
the patient's disease in the preoperative period, but cardiovascular stability
may actually be improved by the persistence of propranolol effects during
anesthesia. The lower heart rate and blood pressure are favorable for mini-
mizing myocardial oxygen demands, and the incidence and severity of episodes of tachycardia and dysrhythmias are probably less in patients maintained on β-blockers up to the time of surgery.

Propranolol should not be abruptly withdrawn, even as early as 10
hours prior to surgery. The question of gradual withdrawal of therapy prior
to surgery has not been well resolved, but in the absence of apparent complications from continued propranolol therapy there is little justification for
even gradual withdrawal.

SUMMARY

In an attempt to resolve the controversy concerning propranolol therapy in
patients undergoing coronary artery revascularization surgery, 54 consecutive patients with stable angina pectoris receiving chronic propranolol therapy entered a randomized trial and were compared with 17 patients on no
propranolol therapy (Group I). The 54 patients were divided into three treatment groups: in Group II (n = 17) propranolol was abruptly withdrawn 48
hours prior to surgery; in Group III (n = 18) propranolol was abruptly withdrawn 10 hours prior to surgery; in Group IV (n = 19) propranolol was main-

tained until the morning of surgery, half the usual dose was given 2 hours prior to surgery, and intravenous propranolol was administered every 4 hours postoperatively. Patients in Groups II and III had significantly higher increases in RPP during intubation and in postoperative periods as compared to Groups I and IV. Group IV had the lowest increase in RPP during intubation and a significantly lower incidence of postoperative supraventricular arrhythmias. Patients abruptly withdrawn from propranolol, at 10 or 48 hours preoperatively are more prone to increments in myocardial oxygen demands than those patients not treated with propranolol postoperatively or maintained on the drug. Plasma renin activity, although lower in patients treated with propranolol (Group IV), did not seem to play a role in the RPP increments seen. The increased sympathetic tone associated with intubation and the postoperative period most likely contribute to the increments in RPP and decreased incidence of arrhythmia. These data show the following: (1) Propranolol may be given safely to patients at the time of coronary artery bypass and maintained postoperatively without a decrement in left ventricular performance. (2) There is a "rebound effect" or increased sympathetic activity in patients who have propranolol abruptly withdrawn 10 or 48 hours prior to surgery. (This "rebound effect" causes a marked increase in myocardial oxygen demands during intubation and the postoperative periods, with an increased incidence of arrhythmias.) (3) Continuous propranolol treatment up until the time of surgery with maintenance of intravenous therapy in the immediate postoperative period provides protection against these complications. (4) The data and implications can reasonably be expected to apply to propranolol treated patients with angina pectoris undergoing general anesthesia and noncardiac surgical procedures.

REFERENCES

1. Frishman W, Silverman R: Clinical pharmacology of the new beta adrenergic blocking ing drugs. Part 3. Comparative clinical experience and new therapeutic applications. Am Heart J 98: 119, 1979
2. Viljoen JF, Estafanous FG, Kellner GA: Propranolol and cardiac surgery. J Thorac Cardiovasc Surg 64: 826, 1972
3. Boudoulas H, Lewis RP, Snyder GL, Karayannacos P, Vasko JS: Beneficial effect of continuation of propranolol through coronary bypass surgery. Clin Cardiol 2: 87–91, 1979
4. Slogoff S, Keats AS, Ott E: Preoperative propranolol therapy and aortocoronary bypass operation. JAMA 240: 1487–1490, 1978
5. Kirsh MM, Behrendt DM, Jackson AP, et al.: Myocardial revascularization in patients receiving long-term propranolol therapy. Ann Thorac Surg 25: 117–121, 1978
6. Romagnoli A, Keats AS: Plasma and atrial propranolol after preoperative withdrawal. Circulation 52: 1123–1127, 1975
7. Alderman EL, Coltart DJ, Wettach GE, Harrison DC: Coronary artery syndromes after sudden propranolol withdrawal. Ann Intern Med 81: 625, 1974
8. Miller RR, Olson HG, Amsterdam EA, Mason DT: Propranolol withdrawal rebound

phenomenon. Exacerbation of coronary events after abrupt cessation of antianginal therapy. N Engl J Med 293: 416–418, 1975

9. Shand DG: Propranolol withdrawal. N Engl J Med 293: 449–450, 1975

10. Caralps JM, Mulet J, Wienke HR, Moran JM, Pifarré R: Results of coronary artery surgery in patients receiving propranolol. J Thorac Cardiovasc Surg 67: 526–529, 1974

11. Moran JM, Mulet J, Caralps JM, Pifarré R: Coronary revascularization in patients receiving propranolol. Circulation 49 + 50 (Suppl II): II-116, 1974

12. Kaplan JA, Dunbar RW: Propranolol and surgical anesthesia. Anes Analg 55: 1–5, 1976

13. Kopriva CJ, Guinazu A, Barash PG: Massive propranolol therapy and uncomplicated cardiac surgery. JAMA 239: 1157–1158, 1978

14. Kopriva CJ, Brown ACD, Pappas G: Hemodynamics during general anesthesia in patients receiving propranolol. Anesthesiology 48: 28–33, 1978

15. Jones EL, Kaplan JA, Dorney ER, King SB, Douglas JS, Hatcher CR: Propranolol therapy in patients undergoing myocardial revascularization. Am J Cardiol 38: 696, 1976

16. Boudoulas H, Snyder GL, Lewis RP, et al.: Safety and efficacy of continued propranolol administration through coronary bypass surgery. Am J Cardiol 41: 359, 1978 (Abs)

17. Kaplan JA, Dunbar RW, Bland JW, Sumpter R, Jones EL: Propranolol and cardiac surgery: a problem for the anesthesiologist. Anes Analg 54: 571, 1975

18. Salazar C, Frishman W, Friedman S, et al.: β-blockade for supraventricular tachycardia post-coronary artery surgery: a propranolol withdrawal syndrome. Angiology 30: 816, 1979

19. Robinson BF: Relation of heart rate and systolic blood pressure to the onset of pain in angina pectoris. Circulation 35: 1072, 1967

20. Nelson RR, Gobel FL, Jorgenson CR, Wang K, Wang Y, Taylor HL: Hemodynamic predictors of myocardial oxygen consumption during static and dynamic exercise. Circulation 50: 1179, 1974

21. Coltart DJ, Shand DG: Plasma propranolol levels in the quantitative assessment of β-adrenergic blockade in man. Br Med J 3: 731, 1970

22. Chervu LR, Lory M, Liang T, Lee HB, Blaufox MD: Determination of plasma renin activity by radioimmunoassay: Comparison of results from two commercial kits with bioassay. J Nucl Med 13: 806, 1972

23. Powell CE, Slater IH: Blocking of inhibitory adrenergic receptors by a dichloro-analog of isoproterenol. J Pharmacol Exp Ther 122: 480, 1958

24. Johnstone M: Propranolol during halothane anesthesia. Br J Anaesth 38: 516, 1966

25. Faulkner SL, Hopkins JT, Boerth RC, et al.: Time required for complete recovery from chronic propranolol therapy. N Engl J Med 289: 607, 1973

26. Shand DG, Wood AJJ: Editorial: Propranolol withdrawal syndrome — why? Circulation 58: 202, 1978

27. Frishman W, Silverman R, Strom J, et al.: Clinical pharmacology of the new beta adrenergic blocking drugs. Part 4. Adverse effects. Choosing a β-adrenoceptor blocker. Am Heart J 98: 256, 1979

28. Frishman WH, Christodoulou J, Weksler B, et al.: Abrupt propranolol withdrawal in angina pectoris: Effects on platelet aggregation and exercise tolerance. Am Heart J 95: 169, 1978

29. Boudoulas H, Lewis RP, Kates RE, Dalamangas G: Hypersensitivity to adrenergic stimulation after propranolol withdrawal in normal subjects. Ann Intern Med 87: 433, 1977

30. Shiroff RA, Mathis J, Zelis R, et al.: Propranolol rebound — a retrospective study. Am J

Cardiol 41: 778, 1978

31. Tomori Z, Widdicombe JG: Muscular bronchomotor and cardiovascular reflexes elicited by mechanical stimulation of the respiratory tract. J Physiol (Lond) 200: 25, 1969

32. Prys-Roberts C, Greene LT, Melache R, Foëx P: Studies of anesthesia in relation to hypertension. II: Haemodynamic consequences of induction and endotracheal intubation. Br J Anaesth 43: 531, 1971

33. Prys-Roberts C, Foëx P, Biro GP, Roberts JG: Studies of anaesthesia in relation to hypertension, V: Adrenergic beta-receptor blockade. Br J Anaesth 45: 671, 1973

34. Stoelting RK, Peterson C: Circulatory changes in patients with coronary artery disease following thiamylal-succinylcholine and tracheal intubation. Anes Analg 55: 232, 1976

35. DeVault M, Greifenstein FE, Harris LC: Circulatory responses to endotracheal intubation in light general anesthesia — the effect of atropine and phentolamine. Anesthesiology 21: 360, 1960

36. Bassell GM, Lin YT, Oka Y, Becker RM, Frater RWM: Circulatory response to tracheal intubation in patients with coronary artery disease and valvular disease. Bull NY Acad Med 54: 842, 1978

37. Boudoulas H, Lewis RP, Vasko JS, Karayannacos PE, Beaver BM: Left ventricular function and adrenergic hyperactivity before and after saphenous vein bypass. Circulation 53: 802, 1976

38. Wallen JL, Kaplan JA, Jones EL: Anesthesia for coronary revascularization. In Kaplan J (ed): Cardiac Anesthesia. New York: Grune and Stratton, 1979, pp 270-271

39. Whelton PK, Flaherty JT, MacAllister NP, et al.: Hypertension following coronary artery bypass surgery: the role of preoperative propranolol therapy. Am J Cardiol 43: 422, 1979 (Abs)

40. Goldstein R, Corash L, Tallman J, et al.: Decrease in platelet survival and enhancement of sympathetically mediated reflex rises in heart rate after abrupt withdrawal of propranolol. Am J Cardiol 43: 416, 1979 (Abs)

41. Bernstein V, Miyagishima RT: Rapid beta blockade for control of atrial arrhythmias following coronary bypass surgery. Ann Roy Coll Phys Surg Can 11: 33, 1978 (Abs)

42. Roberts AJ, Niarchos AP, Subramanian VA, et al.: Systemic hypertension associated with coronary artery bypass surgery: predisposing factors, hemodynamic characteristics, humoral profile, and treatment. J Thorac Cardiovasc Surg 74: 846, 1977

43. Hine IP, Wood WG, Mainwaring B, et al.: The adrenergic response to surgery involving cardiopulmonary bypass, as measured by plasma and urinary catecholamine concentrations. Br J Anaesth 48: 355, 1976

44. Barta E, Kuzela L, Kvetnansky R, Activity of sympathetic nerves in heart during cardiopulmonary bypass in patients. J Cardiovasc Surg 17: 174, 1976

45. Tan CK, Glisson SN, El-Etr AA, Ramakrishnaiak KB: Levels of circulating norepinephrine and epinephrine before, during and after cardiopulmonary bypass in man. J Thorac Cardiovasc Surg 71: 928, 1976

46. Pratilas V, Vlachakis ND, Litwak R: Hypertension and plasma catecholamines following aorto-coronary bypass surgery (abs). Clin Res 25: 244A, 1977

47. Fouad FM, Estafanous FG, Tarazi RC: Hemodynamics of postmyocardial revascularization hypertension. Am J Cardiol 41: 564, 1978

48. Wallach R, Karp RB, Reves LG, Oparil S, James TN: Mechanism of hypertension after saphenous vein bypass surgery (abstr). Circulation (Suppl III) 55,56: III-141, 1977

49. Langou RA, Wiles JC, Peduzzi PN, Hammond GL, Cohen LS: Incidence and mortali-

ty of perioperative myocardial infarction in patients undergoing coronary artery bypass grafting. Circulation (Suppl II) 56: II-54, 1977

50. Taylor KM, Morton IJ, Brown JJ, Bain WH, Caves PK: Hypertension and the renin-angiotensin system following open heart surgery. J Thorac Cardiovasc Surg 74: 839, 1977

51. Niarchos AP, Roberts AJ, Case D, Gay WA, Laragh JH: Hemodynamic characteristics of hypertension after coronary bypass surgery and effects of the converting enzyme inhibitor. Am J Cardiol 43: 586, 1979

52. Wilson M, Morgan G, Morgan T: The effect of blood pressure of β-adrenoceptor-blocking drugs given once daily. Clin Sci Mol Med 51: 527s, 1976

53. Boudoulas H, Beaver BM, Kates RE, Lewis RP: Pharmacodynamics of inotropic and chronotropic responses to oral therapy with propranolol. Chest 73: 146, 1978

54. Frishman W: Clinical pharmacology of the new beta adrenergic blocking drugs. Part 1. Pharmacodynamic and pharmacokinetic properties. Am Heart J 97: 663, 1979

55. Shand DG: Pharmacokinetics of propranolol: a review. Postgrad Med J 52 (Suppl 4): 22, 1976

56. Bristow JO: A cardiologist's view of coronary bypass surgery. In Yu PN, Goodwin JF (eds): Progress in Cardiology, Vol 6. Philadelphia, Lea and Febiger, 1977, pp 28-29

57. Hug CC: Pharmacology — anesthetic drugs. In Kaplan J (ed): Cardiac Anesthesia. New York: Grune & Stratton, 1979, pp 7-13

58. Slogoff S, Keats AS, Hibbs CW, Edmonds CH, Bragg DA: Failure of general anesthesia to potentiate propranolol activity. Anesthesiology 47: 504, 1977

59. Tyras DH, Stothert JC, Kaiser GC, et al.: Supraventricular tachyarrhythmias after myocardial revascularization: a randomized trial of prophylactic digitalization. J Thorac Cardiovasc Surg 77: 310, 1979

60. Isom OW, Spencer FC, Feigenbaum H, Cunningham J, Roe C: Pre-bypass myocardial damage in patients undergoing coronary revascularization: an unrecognized vulnerable period. Circulation 52 (Suppl II): 119, 1975 (abs)

61. Delva E, Maillé JG, Solymoss BC, et al.: Evaluation of myocardial damage during coronary artery grafting with serial determinations of serum CPK MB isoenzyme. J Thorac Cardiovasc Surg 75: 467, 1978

62. Logue RB, Kaplan JA: Medical management in non-cardiac surgery. In Hurst JW (ed): The Heart. New York: McGraw-Hill, 1978, p 1765

63. Scott DB, Buckley FP, Drummond GB, Littlewood DG, MacRae WR: Cardiovascular effects of labetalol during halothane anaesthesia. Br J Clin Pharmacol (Suppl 3) 817, 1976

64. Brichard G: Practolol in anesthesia. Acta Cardiol (Brux) (Suppl) 16: 119, 1972

65. Malcolm-Thomas B, Rolly G: Preliminary report on the use of practolol in anaesthesia. Acta Cardiologica (Brux) (Suppl) 16: 102-108, 1972

66. Yoshikawa K, Tosaki Y, Yoshiya I: Use of LB-46, a new anti-arrhythmic agent, during anesthesia. Med J Osaka Univ 23: 189-197, 1972

67. Nicholas G, Nicholas F, Rozo L: Problems posed by anesthesia in the hypertensive treated with beta-blockers. Arch Mal Coeur 69: 1311-1314, 1976

68. Erding E, Nalbantgil E, Kiliccioglu B, Nalbantgil I, Vidinel I: Prevention by pindolol of electrocardiographic changes during bronchoscopy, performed under local and general anesthesia. Ann Anesthesiol Franc 18: 747-751, 1977

69. Frishman W, Silverman R: Clinical pharmacology of the new beta adrenergic blocking drugs. Part 2. Physiologic and metabolic effects. Am Heart J 97: 797, 1979

CHAPTER SEVEN

Beta-Adrenoceptor Blockade in Myocardial Infarction
THE CONTINUING CONTROVERSY

William H. Frishman

BETA-adrenoceptor blocking drugs have been shown to be safe and effective in the treatment of patients who have hypertension, angina pectoris, hypertrophic cardiomyopathy, thyrotoxicosis, glaucoma, and migraine headaches.[1] The role of these agents in the treatment and prevention of myocardial infarction is controversial, however, due to a lack of adequately controlled clinical trials.

These agents are employed with a view toward improving the quality as well as the quantity of life even though there is no adequate clinical data to prove the latter. The theoretical considerations and clinical experience in the use of β-adrenoceptor blocking drugs during the acute phase of myocardial infarction and for the primary and secondary prevention of acute myocardial infarction and sudden death are assessed in this chapter.

PRIMARY PREVENTION (MYOCARDIAL INFARCTION AND SUDDEN DEATH)

While β-adrenoceptor blockade does not directly affect the progress of coronary atheroma, it does reduce myocardial oxygen requirements.[2] This, in turn, enables the cardiac muscle to tolerate, for a while, what would otherwise be an inadequate supply of oxygen.[2] The reduction of oxygen requirements is due to a decreased heart rate and reduction in myocardial contractility.[3] β-Blockade may improve distribution of flow in the ischemic myocardium[4] as well as improve the utilization of myocardial substrate.[5] These drugs are known to inhibit platelet aggregation[6] and to be potent antiarrhythmic agents.[7]

In patients with angina pectoris, these agents have been useful in reducing pain and improving exercise tolerance.[8] An adequate degree of β-adrenoceptor blockade affords marked relief from pain in 80 percent of cases. This success rate can be improved by selecting the best tolerated β-blocker in combination with nitrates.[9] Thus, the quality of life can be improved in patients with angina pectoris.

A major unresolved question in clinical medicine is whether the β-adrenoceptor blockers can influence the natural course of stable angina pectoris by prolonging the patient's life expectancy and reducing the risk of infarction. There are multiple subgroups of patients with angina pectoris defined by differences in symptomology (stable or unstable), coronary anatomy, left ventricular function, and stress test results. These multiple variables make a proper study design almost untenable. The few poorly designed studies that have been completed have not demonstrated any marked reduction in the annual mortality of patients with stable angina pectoris when compared to results of large epidemiologic studies.[10-14] While patients are treated with β-blockers to increase the quality and quantity of life, only the quality of life has been proven to be enhanced. Nevertheless, β-blockade is the treatment of choice for the symptomatic relief of angina pectoris. As in the case with lipid-lowering and platelet-inhibiting agents, however, only theoretical considerations suggest employing β-blockers as primary prophylactic treatment against myocardial infarction and sudden death. Prospective studies with high-risk individuals are necessary to determine if primary preventive treatment is effective. While no definitive evidence exists for the primary prophylactic benefits of β-adrenoceptor blocking drugs, preliminary data suggest that these drugs may be useful in the secondary prevention of reinfarction and sudden death.[15-17]

β-ADRENOCEPTOR BLOCKER THERAPY IN ACUTE MYOCARDIAL INFARCTION

In patients with acute myocardial infarction, the presence of severe pain, tissue injury, and circulatory disturbances provides important physiologic stresses which trigger an increased sympathoadrenal discharge.[7] This observation is based on evidence derived from several studies of urinary free catecholamine excretion,[18,19] and measurements of plasma catecholamine levels during the early stages of myocardial infarction.[20,21]

An increase in circulating catecholamine levels following myocardial infarction may have an important supportive role in the maintenance of the contractile performance of ischemic areas of the myocardium, as well as enhancing residual nonischemic areas.[7,22] There are two important and potentially deleterious consequences of an increase in sympathetic nervous activity, however.

1. Increased sympathoadrenal discharge may be the cause of serious cardiac arrhythmias after myocardial infarction.[7]
2. The positive inotropic and chronotropic effects of catecholamines lead to an increase in total cardiac work and myocardial oxygen consumption.[23] This may be critical, particularly in areas of ischemia at the border of an infarct in which increased oxygen demands may extend areas of necrosis.[24] Isoproterenol has been shown to impair both performance and metabolism of an ischemic myocardium which suggests that enhanced neuroadrenergic activity may be harmful.[25-27]

β-Blocker drugs have been considered for use in patients with acute myocardial infarction to prevent the undesirable consequences of increased sympathoadrenal discharge.[28,29] These agents favorably influence some of the determinants of myocardial oxygen consumption.[24] On the other hand, β-blockade can have dangerous consequences in some cases of fresh infarction. Impulse formation may be greatly impaired and conduction diminished to a degree that causes cardiac arrest. Furthermore, exacerbation of congestive heart failure due to the elimination of the positive inotropic effect of catecholamines has been a known sequelae of β-blockade.[30]

Antiarrhythmic Effects. The value of β-adrenoceptor blockade in patients with dysrhythmias has been established.[7] Antiarrhythmic efficacy in acute myocardial infarction has not been well-documented, however.

The arrhythmogenic actions of catecholamines have been recognized for over 70 years. Recently, it has been found that removal of sympathetic influences to the heart, by whatever means, will lead to a reduction in the incidence of arrhythmias following experimental coronary occlusion in animals.[31,32] Furthermore, the occurrence of ventricular arrhythmias in experimental infarction was found to be associated with increased levels of catecholamines.[33]

The exposure of ischemic tissue to high levels of catecholamines favor the appearance of multiple reentry pathways and the development of ventricular fibrillation.[33,34] These experimental data suggest that β-blockade would be particularly effective in preventing or aborting arrhythmias in acute myocardial infarction. Experimental studies in dogs with myocardial infarction revealed that pretreatment with β-adrenoceptor blockers prevented or reduced the incidence of malignant ventricular tachyarrhythmias.[35]

Randomized controlled trials comparing propranolol[36-39] and alprenolol[40] to placebo in patients with acute myocardial infarction have not revealed differences in the incidence of mortality or morbidity (heart failure or arrhythmia). These studies have been criticized for failing to measure plasma drug levels and for using a fixed dose regimen rather than titrating the drug to the patient's requirements.

Lemberg et al.[41] reported the first major experience using β-blockers in the elective management of arrhythmias after acute myocardial infarction.[41] These investigators reported favorable results with the elective use of propranolol in 34 patients who had 43 episodes of tachyarrhythmia following an acute myocardial infarction complicated by mild to moderate heart failure. The dosage of propranolol employed in these studies was 0.5 to 0.75 mg intravenously given at 2-minute intervals until sinus rhythm returned or the ventricular rate slowed down to 80 beats per minute. The arrhythmias include examples of atrial fibrillation, atrial flutter, supraventricular tachycardia and ventricular tachycardia, all with ventricular rates over 140 beats per minute. A majority of patients responded to a total intravenous dose of less than 5 mg of propranolol.

Lemberg et al.[42] also investigated the use of alprenolol in acute cardiac arrhythmias in patients with infarction and found the drug to be as effective as propranolol in both supraventricular and ventricular arrhythmias. The average intravenous dose was 9.5 mg (range 2 to 20 mg). Comparable experiences with oxprenolol[43] and practolol[44] have been reported.

β-Adrenoceptor blockers have been proven efficacious in the treatment of many patients with atrial fibrillation, atrial flutter, paroxysmal supraventricular tachycardia, junctional tachycardia, and lidocaine-resistant ventricular arrhythmias. These drugs may be used adjunctively with other antiarrhythmic agents as well as in dc electrocardioversion.[7] Overall, the β-adrenoceptor blocking drugs are more effective in paroxysmal supraventricular tachyarrhythmias than they are for ventricular rhythm disturbances.

The therapeutic efficacy of β-blockade as an antiarrhythmic intervention is well accepted. However, potential side effects must be considered when employing β-blocking drugs. These agents can cause or potentiate congestive heart failure, hypotension, atrioventricular conduction delay, and airway obstruction.[7,45,46] It is for these reasons that the routine prophylactic administration of these drugs to all patients with acute myocardial infarction is not justified without hemodynamic monitoring. When using β-blockers as antiarrhythmic agents in acute myocardial infarction, the deleterious effects of tachyarrhythmias in hemodynamic terms and the benefits of reversion to sinus rhythm or slowing of the rapid ventricular rate must be balanced against the possible cardiovascular depression produced by the drugs themselves.

Whether or not β-adrenoceptor blocking drugs with intrinsic sympathomimetic activity (pindolol, acebutolol, oxprenolol) will provide safer antiarrhythmic alternatives to propranolol has not yet been proven in clinical trials.

Reduction or Containment of Myocardial Infarction. β-Blockers would be used extensively in acute myocardial infarction were it not for their negative inotropic effects; β-adrenergic activity is important for diseased hearts.[39,47,48] The negative inotropism of these drugs is due to anti-adrenergic effects rather than membrane depressing properties.[45,46] The negative inotropic effect of β-blockade is not clinically important without evidence of left ventricular dysfunction.[49-51]

Early clinical studies (prior to 1970) in acute myocardial infarction, where oral propranolol was employed as a prophylactic agent, revealed no clinical benefit.[36-39] After these preliminary results, β-adrenoceptor blockers were not used in myocardial infarction until the 1970s. Their use was suggested when investigators recognized that the development of irreversible left ventricular pump failure was related to the area of damaged myocardium, emphasizing a need to preserve the ischemic myocardium. It is now well established that myocardial infarction is not an all-or-none phenomenon. It has been shown that there is an ischemic region around the initially infarcted area that may not necrose until several hours or days have elapsed.[52-53] It has been demonstrated that reduction of myocardial oxygen requirements will decrease the final size of an infarct and an increase in oxygen requirements will increase the infarct.[24,54,55-57] In dogs with an experimental occlusion of a coronary artery, propranolol will reverse the epicardial ST-segment elevation of the electrocardiogram, changes which are said to reflect a reduction in the predicted size of the myocardial infarction. Of interest is the fact that exogenous catecholamines have been found to have the reverse effect.[58]

In man, Pelides et al.[59] have shown that practolol given within 72 hours of an infarct reduced the precordial ST-segment elevation. These findings were amplified by Mueller et al.[50] who demonstrated a reduction of myocardial hypoxia as estimated by increased lactate uptake in patients (Class I and II, New York Heart Classification) after intravenous propranolol was administered within the first 12 hours of infarction. In the study by Mueller et al.[50] there was no deterioration in clinical left ventricular function.[50] Reductions in cardiac contractility, cardiac index, and myocardial oxygen consumption were associated with improved myocardial metabolism and bioenergetics. Despite these favorable hemodynamic and metabolic findings, the investigators could not demonstrate an absolute decrease in infarct size or an increase in ultimate survival.[50] The difficulties in assessing a reduction in predicted myocardial infarction size are due to problems with the measuring modalities.

Gold et al.[60] recently demonstrated a reduction in ischemic injury (defined by reduction of ST-segment elevation) on the ECG when intravenous propranolol was given during acute myocardial infarction. These effects were less marked, however, in patients with total coronary occlusions. These findings suggest that (1) propranolol may be more effective in subendocardial wall infarction where flow is not completely compromised and, in this case, ischemia may be a more important component than necrosis; (2) propranolol may be less effective in transmural myocardial infarction with more complete cessation of effective flow and where necrosis may greatly overshadow reversible ischemia. Nevertheless, these data suggest that a reduction in myocardial oxygen demand might arrest the stepwise progression of myocardial necrosis.

The results of a study by Cairns et al.[61] demonstrated that propranolol, administered an average of 7.6 hours after acute myocardial infarction in 20 patients, appeared to delay the evolution of infarction.[61] In a randomized double-blind clinical trial by Pitt et al.,[62] propranolol was shown to reduce infarct extension.

The benefit-to-risk ratio must be calculated for each patient prior to the use of β-adrenoceptor blockade in acute myocardial infarction. There are inherent problems with this therapy that must be considered:

1. β-Blockers may increase left ventricular volume and end-diastolic pressure by their negative inotropic effects, especially in severely damaged hearts.[47-49,63,64] By this mechanism, they may increase the oxygen demands of ischemic myocardial tissue. At the same time, the drugs may increase left ventricular end-diastolic pressure and limit an already compromised subendocardial blood flow. These risk factors could easily offset the beneficial reduction in heart rate and blood pressure with β-adrenoceptor blockade.
2. Since patients have varying degrees of sympathetic tone, there is no established β-adrenoceptor blocking dose with any agent.[45,63] One patient might require a dose four times that of another patient to achieve the same β-blocking effect. The drug should also be given intravenously in acute myocardial infarction to achieve its immediate effects, and this might precipitate sudden bradyarrhythmias or conduction abnormalities.[7]
3. Despite the adverse effects of isproterenol recently defined in experimental animals with myocardial infarction,[24,27] heightened sympathetic tone may not be deleterious for all patients. Some patients with a considerable amount of frank necrosis and little ongoing ischemia may need their sympathetic tone to preserve pump function. β-Adrenoceptor blockade could actually worsen cardiac failure in these patients.[22]

The widespread administration of β-blocking agents to patients with myocardial infarction is not indicated unless hemodynamic monitoring is available to assess the benefit-to-risk ratio in any given patient. Where ischemia rather than necrosis is the cause of the pathologic problem, β-blockade is recommended, especially in those patients with preinfarction states ("intermediate syndrome"). By decreasing heart rate, blood pressure, and contractility, β-adrenoceptor blockade reduces ischemia and relieves pain. Left ventricular function, which may be transiently depressed in acute ischemia, generally improves as the ischemia is lessened.[50,65] Once the situation is stabilized medically more definitive measures, including coronary angiography and, when appropriate, coronary artery bypass surgery, may be considered.

Excluding patient contraindications, the recommended dose of propranolol for treatment of acute and prolonged myocardial ischemia is 0.05 to 0.10 mg per kg (lean body weight) administered intravenously at a rate of 1 mg per minute.[50] This should be followed by an oral dose regimen designed to achieve adequate β-adrenoceptor blockade.

The potentially protective properties of propranolol in acute myocardial ischemia in the absence of infarction have been reported by several groups. In a randomized double-blind study of 68 patients with unstable angina, the propranolol-treated patients experienced fewer coronary events than placebo-treated patients.[66] In patients admitted to a coronary care unit because of prolonged ischemic chest pain, a myocardial infarction developed less frequently under long-term treatment with β-blocking drugs; 30 of 90 patients experienced infarction in contrast to 62 of 90 patients who did not receive the drug.[67]

β-Adrenoceptor blocking drugs are indicated when angina pectoris develops after acute myocardial infarction, and in a subgroup of patients with myocardial infarction associated with a hyperkinetic circulatory response (i.e., hypertension, tachycardia) without evidence of left ventricular dysfunction.[68]

The results of experimental and clinical research suggest that β-adrenoceptor blockade can play an important role in the treatment of acute myocardial infarction. This blockade decreases cardiac work and improves perfusion and metabolism of ischemic myocardium. The effectiveness of β-adrenoceptor blocking agents depends primarily upon the functional state of the heart. The more left ventricular function is determined by the mechanical and contractile properties of ischemic areas, the more likely β-adrenoceptor blockade will improve oxygenation of the jeopardized myocardium. However, a deleterious effect can be anticipated when the ventricular performance is primarily determined by frank myocardial necrosis. With careful evaluation of the benefits-to-risk potential in individual patients, β-adrenoceptor blockade can be a useful therapeutic intervention for protecting the ischemic myocardium in acute myocardial infarction.

SECONDARY PREVENTION OF MYOCARDIAL INFARCTION AND SUDDEN DEATH

There is currently a 10 percent mortality rate 1 year following a myocardial infarction,[69,70] and this mortality occurs within 1 hour of the onset of symptoms in approximately half of these cases.[71] A therapeutic goal is to decrease the mortality rate in this group of patients at high risk of sudden death. Ventricular tachyarrhythmis are now considered the most important cause of sudden death in patients who are less than 70 years.

A significant reduction in mortality by continuous treatment with procainamide, quinidine, phenytoin, as well as with other new antiarrhythmic agents, after myocardial infarction, has not been demonstrated in controlled clinical trials.[72,73] Short-term trials using propranolol following acute myocardial infarction have shown conflicting results. Snow[74] first reported a substantial reduction of mortality. He treated 52 patients with 60 mg of propranolol daily for 21 days and compared them to 55 control subjects. The results, while impressive, were not conclusive because it was an open label study without a double-blind control group. Several randomized double-blind studies were then initiated. These included about 250 patients with acute myocardial infarction who received an average of 40 to 80 mg of oral propranolol daily. These controlled studies failed to confirm the findings of Snow.[36-39] There were no significant differences in mortality, shock, heart failure, hypotension, or arrhythmias between the treated and untreated patients.

The first long-term study using a β-blocker also failed to demonstrate a decreased mortality. In this double-blind randomized study by Reynolds and Whitlock[75] (Table 7-1), 78 patients were given 100 mg of alprenolol or placebo, four times daily, for 1 year, following the time of admission to a hospital coronary care unit. This trial may have been of too short a duration and involved too few patients to show a difference.

Two major clinical trials from Sweden, using alprenolol in patients with myocardial infarction, have since been completed.[15,16] Alprenolol was chosen as the β-adrenoceptor blocker for study owing to its moderate intrinsic stimulating action[45] and consequent theoretically reduced risk of causing sinus bradycardia. The objectives of these studies were to investigate whether the incidence of recurrence of infarction, sudden death, and total mortality was influenced in patients treated with a β-blocker.

In the study by Wilhelmsson et al (Table 7-1),[15] patients who had a myocardial infarction were less prone to sudden death if treated with a β-blocking drug. In this small, but well-controlled study, 230 patients who had sustained a myocardial infarction were grouped into four separate risk strata which was determined by the degree of previous myocardial damage. Within each stratum alprenolol (400 mg daily), or placebo, was randomly assigned and administered to patients for over 2 years. Within each stratum, the incidence of nonfatal reinfarction appeared much the same, but the incidence of sudden death and total mortality was reduced significantly in patients receiving alprenolol. These results have been questioned because of the use of a fixed dose regimen and the small sample size analyzed.

In the study by Ahlmark et al.[16] a similar reduction in sudden death was seen in patients treated with alprenolol compared to matched controls.

TABLE 7-1. Reported Efficacy of Long-Term β-Adrenoceptor Blockade in Preventing Reinfarction and Sudden Death

Study	No. of Patients	Duration of study (yr)	Regimen	Nonfatal Reinfarction	Sudden Death	Total Mortality
Reynolds and Whitlock[75]	78	1	Alprenolol (39)	4 } (NS)	2 } (NS)	3 } (NS)
			Placebo (39)	4	1	3
Wilhelmsson et al.[15]	230	2	Alprenolol (114)	16 } (NS)	3 } (p<0.05)	7 } (NS)
			Placebo (116)	18	11	14
Ahlmark et al.[16]	162	2	Alprenolol (69)	4 } (p<0.05)	1 } (p<0.05)	5 } (NS)
			No therapy (93)	15	9	11
International Multicentre[17]	3038	up to 3* (mean in 14 mo)	Practolol (1514)	69 } (p<0.10)	30 } (p<0.02)	47 } (p<0.02)†
			Placebo (1524)	89	52	73

NS—not statistically significant.

*Study had to be terminated because of major toxic effects of practolol.

†Reduction in total cardiac mortality was only significant for patients with previous anterior wall myocardial infarction.

In contrast to the findings of Wilhelmsson et al.,[15] these investigators also reported a reduction in the actual reinfarction rate in patients receiving alprenolol. This single-blind randomized trial was carried out for 2 years in 162 patients who had sustained a myocardial infarction (Table 7-1). Patients received either 100 mg of alprenolol four times daily or no β-blocker. This study has been criticized on the grounds that the patients were randomized before the study was open and the control group was not given placebo.

Alprenolol was well-tolerated in the three trials, as demonstrated by the low patient dropout rate because of drug intolerance.[15,16,75] It was concluded that alprenolol could be administered safely to patients with acute myocardial infarction excluding those patients with conduction disease, active bronchospasm, and congestive heart failure.[16,17]

The largest trial of a β-adrenoceptor blocker to date in patients with myocardial infarction was a double-blind randomized multicenter international study in over 3000 patients, comparing practolol with placebo (Table 7-1).[17] Fixed dose practolol (200 mg twice daily), or placebo, was randomly assigned to patients 1 to 4 weeks after an acute myocardial infarction. Unfortunately, the trial was prematurely terminated after the reports of practolol toxicity emerged. However, 330 actively treated patients and 336 placebo treatments were followed for over 2 years. A significant difference was found in the incidence of sudden death within 2 hours after onset of symptoms: 30 patients in the practolol group compared with 52 in the placebo group. There was also a significant difference in the total number of cardiac deaths. A nonsignficant trend toward reduction in nonfatal reinfarctions, 69 compared with 89, was also found. In this study, the beneficial effects seem to be confined to patients with previous anterior wall myocardial infarcts and low diastolic blood pressures at entry. The study also showed a significant reduction in cardiac arrhythmias and in the incidence of angina pectoris with practolol.

The evidence in favor of a prophylactic or "cardioprotective effect" of β-adrenoceptor blocking drugs in the management of patients following myocardial infarction is persuasive. At least three possible mechanisms of action might be implicated: (1) chronic β-blockade might prevent myocardial infarction by reducing myocardial oxygen demands[3] and/or altering abnormal platelet aggregability[6]; (2) by preventing malignant arrhythmias during the initial phase of an infarction,[7] and (3) by influencing the size of the ischemic area (apart from the antiarrhymic action of the β-blocker) irrespective of whether infarction occurred.[50]

Would one β-blocking agent provide a theoretical advantage over another in patients with acute myocardial infarction? With equal degrees of β-blockade, all the available agents are equally effective in the therapy of hypertension, arrhythmias, and angina pectoris.[1,46] Alprenolol, a noncardioselective agent with membrane-stabilizing activity and intrinsic agonist effects, and practolol, an agent which has cardioselective and agonist activities without membrane depressant effects both appear useful as "cardioprotective" agents. It would appear, therefore, that if β-blockade proved to be an effective treatment modality in patients with myocardial infraction, all the β-blocking drugs could be interchanged with the exception of small differences in side effects.

The observations made with alprenolol and practolol need to be reconfirmed and extended to larger patient populations. There were major methodologic problems with both the alprenolol and practolol trials. Currently, the National Institutes of Health is sponsoring a large multicenter trial (β-Adrenoceptor Blocker Heart Attack Trial: BHAT) evaluating long-term oral propranolol therapy in patients with myocardial infarction. This study was designed to eliminate some of the methodologic problem of previous trials. Patients who meet entry criteria will be randomly assigned to receive placebo and propranolol treatment 5 days after infarction. Propranolol is titrated from 180 to 240 mg daily to achieve effective β-adrenoceptor blockade. Serum levels are being monitored and patients observed for up to 4 years. A patient cohort of over 4000 is being evaluated. The data to be collected include the incidence of sudden death, nonfatal reinfarction, fatal myocardial infarctions (not sudden death), noncardiovascular deaths, arrhythmia, and angina pectoris. A similar multicenter trial comparing metoprolol (a cardioselective agent) with placebo, is now being planned.

These well-controlled studies will undoubtedly yield conclusive results that will lay the current controversy to rest. It is anticipated that β-adrenergic blockade will be proven to be not only safe and effective in the management of ischemic heart disease, but also in the prevention of reinfarction.

CONCLUSION

The results of experimental and clinical research suggest that β-adrenoceptor blockers may play an important role in the prevention and treatment of acute myocardial infarction. They decrease cardiac work and improve myocardial metabolism. The drugs are also effective antiarrhythmic agents.

β-Blockers signficantly reduce the symptoms of angina pectoris, but have not been shown to influence the life span of patients in primary prevention trials. Following acute myocardial infarction, however, there is some evidence suggesting that chronic β-blocker therapy can reduce the incidence of sudden death and reinfarction.

In the treatment of acute myocardial infarction, the effectiveness of β-blockade depends upon the functional state of the heart. The more left ventricular function is determined by the mechanical and contractile properties of ischemic areas, the more likely it is that β-blockade will improve oxygenation of jeopardized myocardium. With careful hemodynamic monitoring, therapeutic benefits and potential hazards can be assessed. The early use of β-adrenoceptor blockade may interrupt the stepwise development of myocardial necrosis, salvage myocardial tissue, and improve immediate mortality, and long-term ventricular function.

Future studies will determine whether β-adrenergic blocking drugs can enhance the quantity of life, as well as the quality of life, in patients who have sustained a myocardial infarction.

REFERENCES

1. Frishman W, Silverman R: Clinical pharmacology of the new beta adrenergic blocking drugs. Part 3. Comparative clinical experience and new therapeutic applications. Am Heart J 98:119, 1979
2. Conolly ME, Kersting F, Dollery CT: The clinical pharmacology of the beta-adrenoceptor blocking drugs. Prog Cardiovasc Dis 19:203, 1976
3. Epstein SE, Robinson BF, Kahler RL, Braunwald E: Effects of beta-adrenergic blockade on the cardiac response to maximal and submaximal exercise in man. J Clin Invest 44:1745, 1965
4. Becker LC, Fortuin NJ, Pitt B: Effect of ischemic and anti-anginal drugs on the distribution of radioactive microspheres in the canine left ventricle. Circ Res 28:263, 1971
5. Opie LH, Thomas M: Propranolol and experimental myocardial infarction substrate effects. Postgrad Med J 52 (Suppl 4):124, 1976
6. Frishman WH, Weksler B, Christodoulou P, Smithen C, Killip T: Reversal of abnormal platelet aggregability and change in exercise tolerance in patients with angina pectoris following oral propranolol. Circulation 50:887, 1974
7. Jewitt DE, Singh BN: The role of β-adrenergic blockade in myocardial infarction. Prog Cardiovasc Dis 16:421, 1974
8. Prichard BNC, Gillam PMS: Assessment of propranolol in angina pectoris. Br Heart J 33:473, 1971
9. Wiener L, Dwyer EM Jr, Cox JW: Hemodynamic effects of nitroglycerin, propranolol, and their combination in coronary heart disease. Circulation 39:623, 1969
10. Amsterdam EA, Wolfson S, Gorlin R: Effect of therapy on survival in angina pectoris. Ann Intern Med 68:1151, 1968
11. Lambert DMD: Long-term survival on beta-receptor blocking drugs in general practice — a three year prospective study. In Burley D, et al. (eds): Hypertension — its natural history and treatment (Int Symp Malta). England, Ciba, 1975, p 283.
12. Russek HI: Prognosis in angina pectoris with optimal medical therapy. In Russek HI (ed): New Horizons in Cardiovascular Practice. Baltimore, University Park Press, 1975
13. Warren SG, Brewer DL, Orgain ES: Long-term propranolol therapy for angina pectoris. Am J Cardiol 37:420, 1976
14. Kannel WB, Feinlab M: Natural history of angina pectoris in the Framingham study. Prognosis and Survival. Am J Cardiol 29:154, 1972

15. Wilhelmsson C, Vedin JA, Wilhelmsen L, Tibblin G, Werkö L: Reduction of sudden deaths after myocardial infarction. Lancet 2:1157, 1974

16. Ahlmark G, Saetre H, Korsgren M: Reduction of sudden deaths after myocardial infarction. Lancet 2:1563, 1974

17. Multicentre International Study: Improvement in prognosis of myocardial infarction by long term beta-adrenoceptor blockade using practolol. Br Med J 1:837, 1976

18. Valori C, Thomas M, Shillingford JP: Free noradrenaline and adrenaline excretion in relation to clinical syndromes following myocardial infarction. Am J Cardiol 20:605, 1967

19. Jewitt DE, Mercer CJ, Reid D, et al.: Free noradrenaline and adrenaline excretion in relation to the development of cardiac arrhythmias and heart failure in patients with acute myocardial infarction. Lancet 1:635, 1969

20. Gazes PC, Richardson JA, Woods EF: Plasma catecholamine concentrations in myocardial infarction and angina pectoris. Circulation 19:657, 1959

21. McDonald L, Baker C, Bray C, McDonald A, Restieaux N: Plasma catecholamines after cardiac infarction. Lancet 2:1021, 1969

22. Frishman WH, Sonnenblick EH: Propranolol therapy in acute myocardial infarction. Cardiovasc Med 2:311, 1977

23. Vasu MA, O'Keefe DD, Kapellakis GZ, Daggett WM, Powell WJ Jr.: Myocardial oxygen consumption and hemodynamic effects of dobutamine, epinephrine, and isoproterenol. Fed Proc 34:435, 1975

24. Maroko PR, Kjekshus JK, Sobel BE, et al.: Factors influencing infarct size following experimental coronary artery occlusions. Circulation 43:67, 1971

25. Gunnar RM, Loeb HS, Pietras RJ, Tobin JR Jr.: Ineffectiveness of isoproterenol in shock due to acute myocardial infarction. JAMA 202:1124, 1967

26. Mueller H, Ayres SM, Fianelli S Jr., et al.: Effect of isoproterenol, 1-norepinephrine and intra-aortic counterpulsation on hemodynamics and myocardial metabolism in shock following acute myocardial infarction. Circulation 43:335, 1972

27. Kirk ES, Hirzel HO, Sonnenblick EH: The relative role of supply and demand in the effect of isoproterenol on infarct size. Circulation 55,56 (Suppl): 3:III-149, 1979

28. Black JW: Drug Responses in Man. London, Little, Brown, 1967, p 121

29. Epstein S, Goldstein R, Redwood DR, Kent KM, Smith ER: The early phase of acute myocardial infarction: pharmacologic aspects of therapy. Ann Intern Med 78:918, 1973

30. Brunner H: The pharmacological basis for the cardioprotective action of beta-blockers. In Gross F (ed): The Cardioprotective Action of Beta-Blockers. Baltimore, University Park Press, 1976, p 11

31. Schaal SF, Wallace AG, Sealy WC: Protective influence of cardiac denervation against arrhythmias of myocardial infarction. Cardiovasc Res 3:241, 1969

32. Ebert PA, Vanderbeck RB, Allgood RJ, Sabiston DC: Effect of chronic cardiac denervation on arrhythmias after coronary artery ligation. Cardiovasc Res 4:141, 1970

33. Ceremuzynski L, Staszewska-Barczak J, Herbaczynsha-Cedro K: Cardiac rhythm disturbances and the release of catecholamines after coronary occlusion in dogs. Cardiovasc Res 3:190, 1969

34. Han J: Mechanisms of ventricular arrhythmias associated with myocardial infarction. Am J Cardiol 24:800, 1969

35. Khan MI, Hamilton JT, Manning GW: Protective effects of beta-adrenoceptor blockade in experimental coronary occlusion in conscious dogs. Am J Cardiol 30:832, 1972

36. Balcon R, Jewitt DE, Davies JPH, Oram S: A controlled trial of propranolol in acute myocardial infarction. Lancet 2:917, 1966
37. Clausen J, Felsby M, Jorgense F, et al.: Absence of prophylactic effect of propranolol in myocardial infarction. Lancet 2:920, 1966
38. Norris RM, Caughey DE, Scott PJ: A trial of propranolol in acute myocardial infarction. Br Med J 2:398, 1968
39. Stephen SA: Unwanted effects of propranolol. Am J Cardiol 18:463, 1966
40. Briant R, Norris RM: Alprenolol in acute myocardial infarction. NZ Med J 71:135, 1970
41. Lemberg L, Castellanos A, Arcebal AG: The use of propranolol in arrhythmias complicating acute myocardial infarction. Am Heart J 80:479, 1970
42. Lemberg L, Arcebal AG, Castellanos A, Slavin D: Use of alprenolol in acute cardiac arrhythmias. Am J Cardiol 30:77, 1972
43. Sandler G, Pistevos AC: Use of oxprenolol in cardiac arrhythmias associated with acute myocardial infarction. Br Med J 1:454, 1971
44. Jewitt DE, Croxson R: Practolol in the management of cardiac dysrhythmias following myocardial infarction and cardiac surgery. Postgrad Med J 47 (Suppl):25, 1971
45. Frishman W: Clinical pharmacology of the new beta adrenergic blocking drugs. Part 1. Pharmacodynamic and pharmacokinetic properties. Am Heart J 97:663, 1979
46. Frishman W, Silverman R: Clinical pharmacology of the new beta adrenergic blocking drugs. Part II. Physiologic and metabolic effects. Am Heart J 97:797, 1979
47. Vogel JHK, Blount SG Jr: Modification of cardiovascular responses by propranolol. Br Heart J 29:310, 1967
48. Epstein SE, Braunwald E: Clinical and hemodynamic appraisal of beta-adrenergic blocking drugs. Ann NY Acad Sci 139:952, 1967
49. Wolk MJ, Scheidt S, Killip T: Heart failure complicating acute myocardial infarction. Circulation 45:1125, 1972
50. Mueller HS, Ayres SM, Religa A, Evans RG: Propranolol in the treatment of acute myocardial infarction: effect on myocardial oxygenation and hemodynamics. Circulation 49:1078, 1974
51. Alderman EL, Coltart DJ, Robinson SC, Harrison DC: Effects of propranolol on left ventricular function and diastolic compliance in man. Circulation 48 (Suppl 4):87, 1973
52. Manning JP, Pensinger RR, Fehn PA: Cardiac alkaline phosphatase activity potassium concentration in dogs with acute myocardial infarction. Cardiovasc Res 2:308–313, 1968
53. Cox JL, McLaughlin VW, Flowers NC, Horan LG: The ischemic zone surrounding acute myocardial infarction. Its morphology as detected by dehydrogenase staining. Am Heart J 76:650, 1968
54. Raab W: The nonvascular metabolic myocardial vulnerability factor in "coronary heart disease". Am Heart J 66:685, 1963
55. Maroko PR, Braunwald E: Modification of myocardial infarction size after coronary occlusion. Ann Intern Med 79:720, 1973
56. Redwood DR, Smith ER, Epstein SE: Coronary artery occlusion in the conscious dog. Effects of alteration in heart rate and arterial pressure on the degree of myocardial ischemia. Circulation 46:323, 1972
57. Shell WE, Sobel BE: Deleterious effects of increased heart rate on infarct size in the conscious dog. Am J Cardiol 31:474, 1973

58. Herbaczynska-Cedro K: The influence of adrenaline secretion on the enzymes in heart muscle after acute coronary occlusion in dogs. Cardiovasc Res 4:168, 1970

59. Pelides LJ, Reid DS, Thomas M, Shillingford SP: Inhibition by beta blockade of the ST segment elevation after acute myocardial infarction in man. Cardiovasc Res 6:295, 1972

60. Gold HK, Leinbach RC, Maroko PR: Propranolol-induced reduction of signs of ischemic injury during acute myocardial infarction. Am J Cardiol 38:689, 1976

61. Cairns JS, Klassen G: Modification of acute myocardial infarction by IV propranolol. Circulation 52 (Suppl 2): 107, 1975

62. Pitt B, Weiss JL, Schulze RA, et al.: Reduction of myocardial infarct extension in man by propranolol. Circulation 54 (Suppl 2):29, 1976

63. Frishman W, Smithen C, Befler B, Kligfield P, Killip T: Non-invasive assessment of clinical response to oral propranolol. Am J Cardiol 35:635, 1975

64. Chidsey C, Vogel J: Adrenergic mechanisms in heart failure. In Katlus AA, Ross G, Hall VE (eds): Cardiovascular Beta Adrenergic Responses. Berkeley: University of California Press, 1970, p 81

65. Haneda T, Lee T, Ganz W: Metabolic effects of propranolol in the ischemic myocardium studied by residual sampling. Circulation (Suppl 4):174, 1973

66. Davies RO, Mizgala HF, Tinmouth AL, Waters DD, Counsell J: Prospective controlled trial of long-term propranolol on acute coronary events in patients with unstable coronary artery disease. Clin Pharmacol Ther 17:232, 1975

67. Fox KM, Chopra MP, Portal RW, Aber CP: Long-term beta-blockade: possible protection from myocardial infarction. Br Med J 1:117, 1975

68. Guazzi M: Beta-blockade in hyperkinetic heart syndrome. In Gross F (ed): The Cardioprotective Action of Beta-Blockers. Baltimore, University Park Press, 1976, p 46

69. Pell S, d'Alonzo CA: Immediate mortality and five year survival of employed men with a first myocardial infarction. N Eng J Med 270:915, 1964

70. Norris RM, Mercier CI: Long-term prognosis following treatment in a coronary care unit. Aust NZ Med 1:31, 1973

71. Romo M: Factors related to sudden deaths in acute ischemic heart disease. Acta Med Scand (Suppl) 547:1, 1973

72. Kosowsky BD, Taylor J, Lown A, Ritchie RF: Long-term use of procainamide following acute myocardial infarction. Circulation 47:1204, 1973

73. Collaborative Group: Phenytoin after recovery from myocardial infarction. Lancet 2: 1055, 1977

74. Snow PJD: Effect of propranolol in myocardial infarction. Lancet 2:551, 1965

75. Reynolds JL, Whitlock RML: Effects of a beta-adrenergic receptor-blocker in myocardial infarction treated for one year from onset. Br Heart J 34:252, 1972

CHAPTER EIGHT

Pindolol (LB-46) Therapy For Supraventricular Arrhythmia
A VIABLE ALTERNATIVE TO PROPRANOLOL IN PATIENTS WITH BRONCHOSPASM

William H. Frishman, Richard Davis, Joel Strom,
Uri Elkayam, Morris Stampfer, and Edmund Sonnenblick

S INCE their introduction as antiarrhythmic agents, β-adrenoceptor blocking drugs have been proven to be effective and safe against supraventricular and ventricular arrhythmias, when administered intravenously and orally. β-Blockade appears to be the main antiarrhythmic mechanism, and it is reasonable to expect that all β-adrenoceptor antagonists will have comparable antiarrhythmic efficacy for a given degree of β-blockade.[1] To date, an undisputed superiority of one β-blocking drug over another in the treatment of arrhythmias has not been clearly demonstrated. Any differences in their overall clinical benefits must therefore be assumed to be related to variations in their associated pharmacologic properties (cardioselectivity, intrinsic sympathomimetic activity).[2]

Propranolol blocks both cardiac (β_1) and smooth muscle (β_2) receptors and can precipitate bronchoconstriction in certain patients.[3,4] Some β-receptor blocking drugs have a degree of selectivity for β_1 receptors as opposed to β_2 receptors, and these drugs are less likely to provoke asthma, although the relative risk is hard to quantify and is almost certainly dependent on the dose used.[5] Thus, low doses of a given agent might produce appreciable cardiac β-receptor blockade with only a minor degree of blockade of smooth muscle receptors; however, in high doses selectivity is lost.[6]

Other β-receptor-blocking drugs have a high degree of intrinsic sympathomimetic activity, and this has been claimed to lessen the risk of bronchospasm.[7] If the newer β-adrenoceptor blocking drugs are to be useful, they should be able, with their other pharmacologic properties, to substitute for propranolol in situations where bronchospasm (and myocardial depression) are potential problems. One of these newer agents, pindolol (LB-46), is noncardioselective and has the greatest intrinsic sympathomimetic activity of the β-blocking agents currently available for clinical use.

This chapter reports the efficacy of pindolol in the treatment of supraventricular arrhythmias in patients with propranolol-induced bronchospasm.

PATIENTS AND METHODS

PATIENTS

Eighteen patients, 11 women and 7 men, were studied. Their average age was 59 years (range 31 to 72). Patients were referred for study by their physicians because of supraventricular tachyarrhythmias (which had been responsive to intravenous and/or oral propranolol) where long-term pharmacologic maintenance was not possible because of propranolol-induced bronchospasm documented by pulmonary spirometric studies. Each patient had a history of either bronchial asthma or chronic obstructive pulmonary disease. All subjects had past histories of episodic wheezing and all demonstrated significant reversibility of airway obstruction. No patient demonstrated active wheezing just prior to initial propranolol administration.

The 18 patients manifested the following arrhythmias: atrial fibrillation or flutter (8 patients), paroxysmal atrial tachycardia (7 patients), junctional tachycardia (2 patients), multifocal atrial tachycardia (1 patient). Associated nonpulmonary medical conditions included hyperthyroidism, arteriosclerotic heart disease, and idiopathic subaortic stenosis. Patients took no other antiarrhythmic medication (including digoxin, quinidine) other than β-adrenoceptor blocking agents throughout the course of the study. Patients with poorly controlled congestive heart failure, myocardial infarction within the preceding 2 months, advanced degrees of heart block, or severe restrictive lung disease were excluded. Patients with life-threatening arrhythmias requiring urgent therapy were also excluded.

Each patient gave written informed consent, and the protocol described below was approved by the Albert Einstein College of Medicine Committee on the Use of Human Subjects in Research.

INTRAVENOUS TREATMENT PROTOCOL

All patients received two doses of intravenous placebo at 5-minute intervals. If there was no antiarrhythmic effect 5 minutes after the second placebo dose,* pindolol was administered intravenously with an initial dose of

0.4 mg. This was followed by 0.2 mg every 5 minutes as necessary until the desired response was achieved. The total dose of pindolol never exceeded 1.4 mg per 24 hours. Continuous electrocardiographic monitoring was carried out and blood pressure measured frequently throughout the period of administration. If, after a total dose of 1.4 mg pindolol IV no antiarrhythmic effect was observed, the drug was discontinued.

ORAL TREATMENT PROTOCOL

In order to enter the oral treatment phase of the study, the desired antiarrhythmic response must have been obtained with the intravenous form. Patients who qualified were started on 2.5 mg oral pindolol every 6 hours and titrated to a dose ranging up to 10 mg (orally) every 6 hours. The maintenance dose was established as that regimen which would sustain patients with paroxysmal supraventricular tachycardias in normal sinus rhythm, and patients with atrial fibrillation or flutter, in either normal sinus rhythm or with ventricular rates of less than 100 beats per minute. If patients had a recurrence of their arrhythmia during the oral treatment phase, they could be treated with intravenous pindolol and, if responsive, continued on a higher oral dose. Those patients whose arrhythmias could not be controlled with up to 10 mg PO at 6-hour intervals despite repeated success with intravenous retreatment, were considered nonresponders to oral pindolol.

In the oral pindolol phase (2 months), patients were seen as outpatients and were followed with weekly 24-hour Holter ECG recordings using an Avionics #445 recorder and an Avionics Dynamic Electrocardioscanner #660 A (120 times real time). Patients were also followed with complete blood counts, urinalyses, blood chemistries, chest roentgenograms, and pulmonary function tests (see below).

PULMONARY FUNCTION TESTS

Spirometric determinations of vital capacity (VC) and forced expiratory volume in one second ($FEV_{1.0}$) were made in 9 patients: (1) during a period when patients were not wheezing and were receiving no β-adrenergic-blocking drugs; (2) during propranolol therapy with active wheezing; (3) after propranolol withdrawal. Measurements made in the same patients were taken during the acute intravenous pindolol phase and again during the long-term oral pindolol phase of the study.

*For paroxysmal supraventricular tachycardias, defined as electrocardiographic conversion to normal sinus rhythm; for atrial flutter and fibrillation, conversion to normal sinus rhythm or slowing of the ventricular rate to less than 100 beats per minute for arterial flutter and fibrillation.

Spirometric determinations were made using a Godart Pulmotest Apparatus. Percent differences in mean $FEV_{1.0}/VC$ for the different treatment intervals were tested for significance by the one-sample t-test.

RESULTS

INTRAVENOUS STUDIES

All 18 patients with paroxysmal supraventricular arrhythmia failed to respond to intravenous placebo and received intravenous pindolol (0.4 to 1.4 mg).

Six of seven patients with paroxysmal supraventricular tachycardia converted to normal sinus rhythm. In the six patients with atrial fibrillation, three converted to normal sinus rhythm, and three demonstrated only ventricular rate slowing. Of the two patients with atrial flutter, one converted to normal sinus rhythm, and one had no response. Both patients with junctional tachycardia converted to normal sinus rhythm as did the one patient with multifocal atrial tachycardia (Table 8-1).

TABLE 8-1.   Summary of the Effects of Intravenous Pindolol (LB-46) in the Acute Management of Patients with Supraventricular Tachycardia

	No. of Patients	Ventricular Rate Reduced to 100 Beats/Min with or Without Return to Sinus Rhythm	Return to Sinus Rhythm	No Response
Paroxysmal Supraventricular Tachycardia	7	6	6	1
Atrial Fibrillation	6	6	3	0
Atrial Flutter	2	1	1	1
Junctional Tachycardia	2	2	2	0
Multifocal Atrial Tachycardia	1	1	1	0

Untoward bradyarrhythmias were not observed in any patients. Seventeen of the 18 patients noted no subjective aggravation of their bronchospastic disease; one patient reported a worsening of his asthma. None developed clinical evidence of congestive heart failure.

ORAL STUDIES

The 16 patients who responded to intravenous pindolol therapy received oral therapy (2.5 to 10 mg every 6 hours) for long-term maintenance. Of the six patients with paroxysmal supraventricular tachycardia treated with oral pindolol, four were maintained in normal sinus rhythm (one of these responded well after a second intravenous pindolol intervention). Two patients with paroxysmal supraventricular tachycardia had frequent recurrence of the arrhythmia and were considered nonresponders to oral pindolol. Of the six patients with atrial fibrillation, five continued to respond (with either continued ventricular rate slowing or maintenance in normal sinus rhythm), and one patient reverted to atrial fibrillation with a rapid ventricular response. The patient with multifocal atrial tachycardia could not be maintained in normal sinus rhythm with oral pindolol. The two patients with junctional tachycardia, and the one with atrial flutter, remained in normal sinus rhythm with oral pindolol (Table 8-2).

TABLE 8-2. Summary of the Effects of Oral Pindolol (LB-46) in the Long-Term Management of Patients with Supraventricular Tachycardia

	No. of Patients	Long-Term Efficacy (Rate Slowing or Maintenance in NSR)	Frequent Recurrence of Arrhythmia
Paroxysmal Supraventricular Tachycardia	6	4	2
Atrial Fibrillation	6	5	1
Atrial Flutter	1	1	0
Junctional Tachycardia	2	2	0
Multifocal Atrial Tachycardia	1	0	1

Of the 16 patients receiving oral pindolol therapy, 14 noted no aggravation of their bronchospastic disease, one felt improved, and one experienced an exacerbation. Two patients developed a self-limited morbilliform erythematous rash which did not warrant cessation of drug therapy. One patient complained of transient dizziness without hypotension or bradycardia. There was no subjective or clinical evidence of congestive heart failure in any patient.

PULMONARY FUNCTION STUDIES (FIG. 8-1)

Nine of the patients with propranolol-induced bronchospasm had spirometric measurements performed while on propranolol and again during the pindolol study.

There was a mean 13.2 percent decrease in $FEV_{1.0}/VC$ during propranolol therapy compared to a nontreatment period ($p < 0.01$). Following propranolol withdrawal, $FEV_{1.0}/VC$ increased by a mean of 14.1 percent, ($p < 0.01$), and did not differ significantly from control.

Compared to the prepropranolol and postpropranolol $FEV_{1.0}/VC$ there was essentially no change in $FEV_{1.0}/VC$ with either intravenous or long-term pindolol therapy.

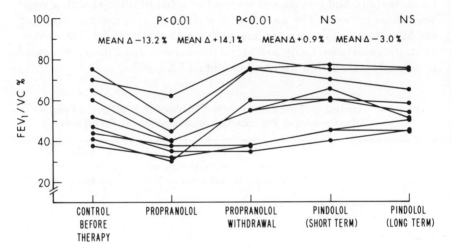

Figure 8-1.   Effects of propranolol and pindolol on $FEV_{1.0}/VC$ in patients with histories of bronchospastic disease aggravated by propranolol. There was a signficant deterioration of $FEV_{1.0}/VC$ with propranolol compared to a nontreatment period, an effect which was completely reversed by drug withdrawal. No significant deterioration in $FEV_{1.0}/VC$ was observed with pindolol treatment in either intravenous or oral form compared to the nontreatment period.

DISCUSSION

β-Adrenergic blockade has become an increasingly popular mode of treatment for supraventricular tachyarrhythmias. In the first three chapters, the newer β-blockers were shown to be as effective as propranolol at a similar degree of β-blockade.[8-10] If these new compounds are to be uniquely useful, they should be able, with their other pharmacologic properties, to substitute for propranolol in situations where bronchospasm, intermittent claudication, or myocardial depression are potential problems.

Propranolol blocks both cardiac (β_1) and smooth muscle (β_2) receptors and, as confirmed by this study, may aggravate bronchospasm in susceptible patients (β_2-receptor blockade). Some β-adrenoceptor blocking drugs have a degree of selectivity for β_1-receptors (as opposed to β_2), and are said to lessen the frequency of bronchospasm in patients with asthma.[11] The drugs with cardioselectivity included practolol and tolamolol (currently under scrutiny because of potentially serious adverse effects), metoprolol (recently approved by the FDA for use in hypertension), acebutolol, and atenolol.[8] These compounds differ from propranolol by a substitution at the paraposition of the aromatic ring. The cardioselectivity of these agents is not absolute and at higher doses (within the therapeutic dose range) β_2 antagonism becomes apparent with the loss of the potential benefit of bronchoprotection.[6]

Other β-receptor blocking drugs have a high degree of intrinsic sympathomimetic activity, a property which has been claimed to lessen the risk of bronchospasm and congestive heart failure. Although β-blockers, by definition, antagonize the actions of agonists, some may paradoxically retain a degree of agonist activity with respect to the same receptor (intrinsic sympathomimetic activity). Initially this property was thought to limit the clinical usefulness of certain β-blockers (practolol, acebutolol, oxprenolol, alprenolol, and pindolol).[12] However, clinical studies have not substantiated this claim and there is no evidence that β-blockers devoid of this effect (propranolol, sotalol, timolol, metoprolol, and atenolol) are more clinically efficacious.

Pindolol (prindolol, LB-46) is, mg for mg, the most potent β-blocker currently available[8,13] and also has the most intrinsic sympathomimetic activity.[8] The drug possesses membrane-stabilizing properties similar to those of propranolol. During the initial clinical trials with pindolol, the drug was thought to be cardioselective because it failed to precipitate bronchospasm in patients.[14] However, increased affinity for the β_1-receptor was shown not to be the cause of this selectivity, and the intrinsic sympathomimetic effects of pindolol on bronchial smooth muscle (i.e., bronchodilatory) may have contributed to its beneficial effects in asthma.[14] If intrinsic sympathomimetic activity of β-adrenergic blockers does play a role in bronchoprotection, this property would be more advantageous than cardioselectivity, since intrinsic sympathomimetic activity is manifested at all dose levels whereas cardioselectivity is only manifested at the lower dose ranges.[6,14]

The results of this study demonstrate that pindolol (used both IV and PO) is a reasonable substitute for propranolol in therapy of patients with supraventricular arrhythmias and bronchospastic disease. Subjectively, 16 of the 18 patients with bronchospasm previously induced by propranolol, noted *no* aggravation of their wheezing with either intravenous or oral pindolol therapy. Objectively, patients treated with pindolol showed no deterioration in $FEV_{1.0}/VC$ on average compared to control, whereas the same patients previously treated with propranolol had showed a marked deterioration in this lung function parameter. Since pindolol does not exhibit cardio-selectivity,[8] one must implicate its intrinsic sympathomimetic activity as the cause of the bronchoprotective effect seen in most of these patients.

Other investigators have reported similar results. In a large series, by Beumer and Hardunk,[7] comparing pulmonary function in patients following treatment with propranolol, pindolol, practolol, alprenolol, and oxprenolol, only practolol and pindolol were found to be bronchoprotective.

Used as antiarrhythmic agents, all β-blocking drugs manifest their action through β-blocking activity, and not through "quinidine-line" membrane depressant activity as was initially proposed.[1] Nevertheless, intrinsic sympathomimetic activity does not appear to interfere with clinical usefulness since multiple trials have shown pindolol to be as effective an antiarrhythmic agent as propranolol.[13,15] In this study, 16 out of 18 patients with supraventricular tachyarrhythmias responded to intravenous pindolol compared to none of the 18 with placebo, and long-term antiarrhythmic benefit was maintained in 12 out of 16 patients with oral pindolol treatment. These patients had had similar antiarrhythmic results with propranolol but could not tolerate the drug because of bronchospasm. Thus, judging from its antiarrhythmic effectiveness alone, pindolol appears to be a reasonable alternative to propranolol.

One might postulate that pindolol would be superior to propranolol where bronchospasm was itself aggravating the arrhythmia. Another potential advantage of pindolol over propranolol might be seen in patients exhibiting "sick sinus syndrome" with a "brady-tachy" presentation. Once the tachyarrhythmia is eliminated, propranolol may further depress the disease sinus node, resulting in a profound bradyarrhythmia. Pindolol, with its intrinsic sympathomimetic activity, does not depress the sinus and atrioventricular node to the same degree as propranolol and may be better tolerated in patients with underlying conduction disease.[16]

Extensive clinical trials using pindolol as an antiarrhythmic agent have been performed in Europe,[17] South Africa, and Japan.[18] The only previous North American experience with pindolol in cardiac arrhythmias was reported by Aronow and Ureyama.[19] These investigators treated 30 patients with supraventricular and ventricular arrhythmias who had no evidence of obstructive lung disease or congestive heart failure. They found the intravenous drug to be extremely useful in atrial fibrillation (conversion to normal sinus rhythm and/or significant ventricular rate slowing), atrial flutter, paroxysmal atrial tachycardia, sinus tachycardia, ventricular tachycardia, and digitalis-induced arrhythmias. Congestive heart failure was precipitated in only one patient.

In studies comparing pindolol with other β-blockers, the drug was shown to be as efficacious as propranolol, practolol, and alprenolol for the treatment of supraventricular arrhythmias.[15]

CONCLUSIONS

Ideally, β-adrenoceptor blocking drugs should be avoided in patients with active bronchospastic disease. However, pindolol (with its intrinsic sympathomimetic properties) may offer an effective alternative to propranolol in situations where a β-blocker is indicated. Whether or not the intrinsic sympathomimetic property of pindolol can protect patients with myocardial depression from further deterioration in their functional status has yet to be determined.

SUMMARY

Pindolol (LB-46) is a new β-adrenoceptor blocking agent with intrinsic sympathomimetic activity. In order to evaluate the efficacy of pindolol in the treatment of patients with supraventricular arrhythmias and a history of propranolol-induced bronchospasm, 18 patients with paroxysmal supraventricular tachycardia, atrial fibrillation, atrial flutter, multifocal atrial tachycardia or junctional tachycardia, were treated with placebo followed by pindolol in intravenous and then oral form. Following a no response placebo period (in all patients), intravenous pindolol converted six of seven patients with paroxysmal supraventricular tachycardia to normal sinus rhythm. In six patients with atrial fibrillation, three reverted to normal sinus rhythm, and three remained in atrial fibrillation but with a slower ventricular response (less than 100 beats per minute). Of two patients with atrial flutter, one converted to normal sinus rhythm, while the other patient failed to respond. Both patients with junctional tachycardia and one with multifocal atrial tachycardia converted to normal sinus rhythm. Long-term oral pindolol therapy sustained these responses in most patients, as documented by serial Holter ECG studies. There was no deterioration in indices of airway resistance ($FEV_{1.0}/VC$) in patients treated with pindolol (both IV and PO), in contrast to a marked deterioration in $FEV_{1.0}/VC$ in the same patients treated with propranolol. Pindolol appears to be a reasonable substitute for propranolol in patients with bronchospastic illness who require β-blockade for control of supraventricular arrhythmias.

REFERENCES

1. Singh BN, Jewitt DE: β-adrenoceptor blocking drugs in cardiac arrhythmias. In Avery G (ed): Cardiovascular Drugs, Vol 2. Baltimore, University Park Press, 1978, p 124
2. Gibson DG: Pharmacodynamic properties of beta-adrenergic receptor blocking drugs in man. Drugs 7: 8-30, 1974

3. Richardson PS, Sterling GM: Effects of β-adrenergic receptor blockade in airway conductance and lung volume in normal and asthmatic subjects. Br Med J 3:143-145, 1969
4. Macdonald AG, Ingram CG, Mc Neill RS: The effects of propranolol on airway resistance. Br J Anaesth 39:919-926, 1967
5. Bernecker C, Ruetscher I: The beta-blocking effect of practolol in asthmatics. Lancet 2:662, 1970
6. Lertora JL, Mark AL, Johannsen VJ, Wilson WR, Abboud F: Selective beta-1 receptor blockade with oral practolol in man. J Clin Invest 56:719-724, 1975
7. Beumer HM, Hardunk HJ: Effects of beta-adrenergic blocking drugs on ventilatory function in asthmatics. Eur J Clin Pharm 5:77-80, 1972
8. Frishman W: Clinical Pharmacology of the new beta adrenergic blocking drugs (part 1): Pharmacodynamic and pharmacokinetic properties. Am Heart J 97:663-670, 1979
9. Frishman, W, Silverman R: Clinical pharmacology of the new beta adrenergic blocking drugs (part 2): Physiologic and metabolic effects. Am Heart J 97: 797-807, 1979
10. Frishman W, Silverman R: Comparative clinical experience and new therapeutic applications (part 3). Am Heart J 98: 119-131, 1979
11. Fitzgerald JD: Cardioselective beta adrenergic blockage. Proc Royal Soc Med 65:761-764, 1972
12. Waal-Manning H, Simpson FO: Paradoxical effect of pindolol. Br Med J 3:155-156, 1975
13. Arbab AG, Hicks DC, Turner P: Relative potency of intravenous prindolol and propranolol in man. Br J Pharmacol 42:655-666, 1971
14. Imhof PR: Characterization of beta blockers as anti-hypertensive agents in the light of human pharmacology studies. In Schweizer W (ed): Beta-Blockers — Present Status and Future Properties. Bern, Huber, 1974 pp 40-50
15. Levi GF, Proto C: Combined treatment of atrial fibrillation with quinidine and beta-blockers. Br Heart J 34:911-914, 1972
16. Giudicelli JF, Lhoste F, Bossier JR: β-adrenergic blockade and atrio-ventricular conduction impairment. Eur J Pharmacol 31:216-225, 1975
17. Storstein L: LB-46, A new β-adrenergic blocking agent in cardiac arrhythmias. Acta Med Scand 191:423-428, 1972
18. Kimura E: Some clinical aspects of the effects of beta-blocking agents especially LB-46. New Horizons Med 1:85-88, 1970
19. Aronow WS, Uyeyama RR: Treatment of arrhythmias with pindolol. Clin Pharmacol Ther 13:15-22, 1972

CHAPTER NINE

Comparison of Pindolol and Propranolol in Treatment of Patients with Angina Pectoris

THE ROLE OF INTRINSIC SYMPATHOMIMETIC ACTIVITY

William H. Frishman, John Kostis, Joel Strom,
Maryhelen Hossler, Uri Elkayam, Susan Goldner,
Richard Davis, Jerome Weinstein, and
Edmund Sonnenblick

THE sympathetic nervous system, through its β-adrenergic actions, markedly influences myocardial oxygen requirements by accelerating the heart rate and enhancing myocardial contractility. A major advance in the symptomatic treatment of angina pectoris occurred with the clinical introduction of β-adrenergic blocking agents which could block these sympathetically mediated effects.[1]

Four main factors influence oxygen demand by the left ventricle: heart rate, ventricular systolic pressure, rate of rise of left ventricular pressure (speed of left ventricular contraction), and the size of the left ventricle.[2]

Heart rate and systolic pressure seem the most important since it has been shown that their product in any individual with typical angina pectoris tends to be the same whether angina occurs spontaneously or is precipitated by exercise.[3] All β-blocking drugs reduce the increment in heart rate with exercise and allow a longer time for diastolic filling. β-Blockade also reduces the rise of blood pressure on exercise, the velocity of cardiac contraction, and oxygen consumption at any given workload.[4,5] When myocardial oxygen requirements are decreased, increased exercise tolerance and decreased frequency of angina attacks result. β-Blocking drugs have other actions (on platelets and metabolism) which may play a part in their antianginal action.[6,7]

Propranolol, a β-adrenoceptor blocker, has been proven effective in many patients with angina pectoris. The drug is a nonselective β-blocker with membrane depressant effects and no intrinsic sympathomimetic activity. The drug is contraindicated in patients with active asthma and congestive heart failure, conditions which can be aggravated by propranolol.[8-11]

Pindolol is a new β-adrenoceptor blocker with the most pronounced intrinsic sympathomimetic activity (partial agonist property) of β-blocking agents currently available.[12] As a β-blocker it is four or five times more potent (mg for mg) than propranolol,[8] and has been shown to be an effective antiarrhythmic,[13,14] antihypertensive,[15] and antianginal agent.[16] It is still debated, however, whether the presence of intrinsic sympathomimetic activity constitutes an advantage or disadvantage in cardiac therapy. It has been claimed by some investigators that intrinsic sympathomimetic activity protects against cardiac failure,[17] severe bradycardia,[18] and bronchial asthma.[19,20] On the other hand, other investigators believe that intrinsic sympathomimetic activity may partially negate the therapeutic benefit of β-adrenergic blockade.[21,22]

The purpose of this study was to compare the clinical effectiveness of two β-blocking agents: pindolol, a drug with intrinsic sympathomimetic activity, and propranolol, a drug lacking this property, in patients with angina pectoris. The effects of the two drugs were compared on the following parameters: (1) angina attack frequency; (2) exercise tolerance measured by treadmill testing; and (3) left ventricular function measured by echocardiography. Also studied were the comparative effects of gradual drug withdrawal in patients after chronic therapy.

METHODS

PATIENTS

Forty-one patients with angina pectoris due to ischemic coronary artery disease were studied. There were 35 male and 6 female patients; the average age was 55 years (range 38 to 78 years). The diagnosis of coronary disease was established by coronary angiography in 33 patients (a stenosis compromising the lumen of at least one major coronary artery by more than 75 percent), or by a previously documented myocardial infarction (appearance of new pathologic ECG Q waves, compatible clinical history and elevation of SGOT and CPK to at least twice the normal values). In addition, every patient had a positive treadmill exercise test showing at least a 1-mm ECG ST-segment ischemic type depression, in association with typical angina pectoris pain.

Additional criteria for inclusion were: (1) at least five attacks of angina pectoris for 2 weeks for 3 months with no evidence for an accelerated course; and, (2) absence of coexistent valvular heart disease, congestive heart failure, hypertension, bronchial asthma requiring continued treatment with bronchodilators, severe bradycardia (resting heart rate 50 beats per minute), intermittent claudication, and either myocardial infarction or a coronary artery bypass within 3 months.

The patients received no drug therapy other than sublingual nitroglycerin and the study medications. Informed consent was obtained in all instances.

EXPERIMENTAL DESIGN

The study was divided into three periods: (1) A 4-week, run-in period during which all patients took propranolol, 10 mg orally, four times a day, in single-blind fashion. (2) Randomization in double-blind fashion was then carried out with patients divided into two treatment groups (8 weeks). The first group (n = 23) received pindolol in increasing oral doses: 2.5 mg four times a day for 2 weeks, 5 mg four times a day for 2 weeks, 10 mg four times a day for 4 weeks. The second treatment group (n = 18) received oral propranolol: 10 mg four times a day for 2 weeks, 20 mg four times a day for 2 weeks, and 40 mg four times a day for 4 weeks. (3) At the end of the last 4-week treatment interval, the medications were gradually tapered (double blind) to 0 over a period of 2 weeks using the following regimen:

Days 1–4	Pindolol 5.0 mg qid; propranolol 20 mg qid
Days 5–8	Pindolol 2.5 mg qid; propranolol 10 mg qid
Days 9–12	Pindolol 2.5 mg bid; propranolol 10 mg bid
Days 13–14	Pindolol 2.5 mg QD; propranolol 10 mg QD

METHODS OF OBSERVATION

All patients kept a detailed daily record of the angina attacks they experienced, the number of nitroglycerin tablets taken, and an estimation of the physical activity for that day. Every 2 weeks the patients were evaluated with a detailed history and physical examination, and two treadmill exercise tests were performed 15 minutes apart. The second exercise test was used for analysis. Sixteen patients underwent serial resting echocardiographic studies at 2-week intervals. Complete blood counts, uninalyses, chest roentgenograms, resting electrocardiograms, determinations of serum antinuclear antibody, and biochemical blood screens (total protein, albumin, calcium, phosphate, cholesterol, uric acid and blood urea nitrogen, glucose, sodium, potassium, total bilirubin, alkaline phosphatase, SGOT, SGPT,

CPK, LDH, CO_2, chloride) were performed at entry, at the end of the run-in period, and at the end of the treatment interval.

EXERCISE TESTS

Multistage exercise testing was performed with the use of a treadmill. Patients were studied biweekly with duplicate studies in the postabsorptive period according to the following protocol:

At 1 mile per hour at 0° elevation for 3 minutes
At 1 mile per hour at 10 percent grade for 3 minutes
At 1.5 miles per hour at 10 percent grade for 3 minutes
At 2 miles per hour at 12 percent grade for 3 minutes
At 3.0 miles per hour at 15 percent grade for 3 minutes (9 mets)
At 3.0 miles per hour at 17 percent grade for 3 minutes
At 3.4 miles per hour at 20 percent grade for 3 minutes (13 mets)
At 4 miles per hour at 22 percent grade for 3 minutes
At 4.5 miles per hour at 24 percent grade for 3 minutes
At 5 miles per hour at 26 percent grade for 3 minutes

The blood pressure was measured every 3 minutes by the auscultatory method and the ECG monitored on the oscilloscope. The end-point of exercise was angina pectoris defined by the patient's typical and characteristic chest pain discomfort. Several patients receiving β-blockers did not develop angina and were forced to stop because of excessive fatigue. An abnormal electrocardiographic response was defined as a flat or down-sloping ST-segment depression of 1 mm of 0.08 seconds duration, after the terminus of the QRS complex, with the P-Ta segment as the baseline of reference.

Work performance was expressed in mets correlating with the level of exercise achieved on the treadmill. The product of heart rate and systolic blood pressure, an indirect index of myocardial oxygen consumption,[3] was calculated from measurements obtained at the exact end-point of exercise.

ECHOCARDIOGRAMS

Serial echocardiographic studies were obtained in 16 cases, just before exercise testing, with the patient in the supine position. A Hoffrel 101 C echocardiograph, with a 2.25 mHz transducer focused at 7.5 cm, was used.

Minor axis end-diastolic dimension was measured at the point where posterior wall endocardium and septum were maximally separated, and end-systolic dimension at the point where they approached each other maximally. The left ventricular dimensions, measured by ultrasound, have been found to approximate closely the left ventricular minor axis in the anteroposterior projection, both at end-diastole and end-systole. The heart was assumed to be a sphere for calculation of left ventricular volume. End-diastolic and end-systolic volumes were calculated as the cube function of the minor axis end-diastolic and end-systolic diameters, respectively. Ejection fraction was obtained by subtracting end-systolic from end-diastolic volume and dividing this value by the end-diastolic volume. In all instances, several cardiac cycles were analyzed and mean values calculated. This method is limited by the inability of the ultrasonic beam to scan the entire ventricle so that only a limited portion of this chamber can be examined. Consequently, the performance of nonvisualized areas is unknown and this may lead to inaccuracies of the technique in patients with left ventricular asynergy.[23] In selected patients, however, determinations of volume and ejection fraction have proven valuable, particularly when serial measurements are made in the same patient.[24-26]

STATISTICAL ANALYSIS

Group means are presented with the standard error of the mean as the index of depression. Results were entered into an IBM 370/168 computer and analyzed using the SPSS statistical package. Differences were calculated by two-way analysis of variance.

RESULTS (Table 9-1)

EFFECTS ON ANGINA ATTACK FREQUENCY (Fig. 9-1)

At the peak pindolol dose (10 mg every 6 hours), the mean number of angina pectoris attacks every 2 weeks decreased from 18.4 ± 2.8 during the run-in period to 10.7 ± 2.2, ($p < 0.01$). At the peak propranolol dose (40 mg

TABLE 9-1.   The Effects of Pindolol and Propranolol
on Hemodynamic Functions and Exercise Tolerance

	Pindolol	Propranolol
Resting heart rate	↔	↓
Resting blood pressure	↓↔	↓↔
Resting double product	↓	↓↓
Rate of heart rate increase with exercise	↓	↓
Rate of systolic blood pressure increase with exercise	↓	↓
Rate of HR × BP increase with exercise	↓	↓
Resting ejection fraction (echo)	↔	↓
Resting end-diastolic volume (echo)	↑↔	↑
Exercise tolerance	↑	↑

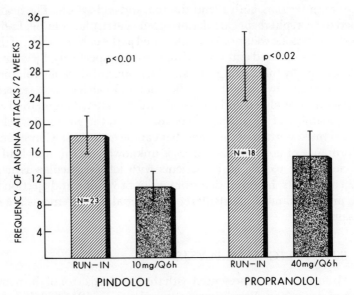

Figure 9-1. A significant decrease in the frequency of anginal attacks in 2 weeks is seen with both pindolol 40 mg per day and propranolol 160 mg per day compared to the run-in period. There was no significant difference in the effectiveness of the two drugs in reducing the frequency of angina attacks.

every six hours), the biweekly attack frequency decreased from 28.5 +5.1 to 15.1+3.6 (p < 0.02). A differential effect of propranolol and pindolol on the reduction in frequency of anginal attacks every 2 weeks was not observed when the data were analyzed by analysis of variance. Thus, pindolol and propranolol (in the doses used) are equally effective in the symptomatic relief of patients with angina pectoris.

During the active treatment phase of the study no patient had an exacerbation of his or her angina attack frequency.

EFFECTS OF PINDOLOL AND PROPRANOLOL ON RESTING HEART RATE, BLOOD PRESSURE, AND DOUBLE PRODUCT (HR×BP) (Figs. 9-2, 9-3, 9-4, Table 9-1)

At peak dose, propranolol decreased the resting heart rate from 70.5 ±2.2 to 62.2 ±2.4 beats per minutes (p < 0.01). The systolic blood pressure decreased from 123.5 ±3.7 to 116.8 ±3.5 mm Hg. Similarly, the HR × BP decreased from 8677 ±423 to 7338 ±455 mm Hg·min^{-1}, (p < 0.005). In contrast, pindolol, at peak dose, did not appreciably decrease the resting heart rate, 66.8 ±1.9 to 64.6 ±1.2 beats per minute, P = NS. The systolic blood pressure decreased slightly from 122.0 ±3.3 to 118 ±19 mm Hg. A

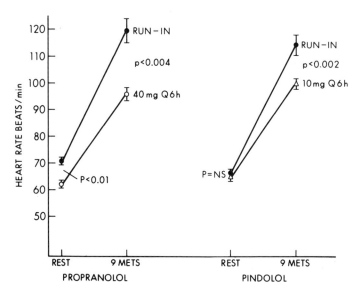

Figure 9-2. Effects of pindolol and propranolol on the heart rate at rest and during exercise (9 mets). A significant decrease in the resting heart rate and the heart rate increment with exercise is seen with propranolol (160 mg per day) compared to the run-in period. There is no change in the resting heart rate in patients treated with pindolol (40 mg per day), however, the heart rate increment with exercise is significantly blunted.

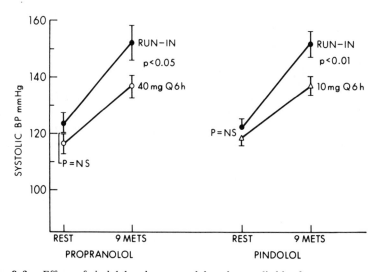

Figure 9-3. Effects of pindolol and propranolol on the systolic blood pressure at rest and during exercise (9 mets). There is a slight but insignificant drop in systolic blood pressure seen with both pindolol and propranolol compared to the run-in period. The systolic blood pressure increment with exercise is similarly blunted in both pindolol- and propranolol-treated patients compared to the run-in period.

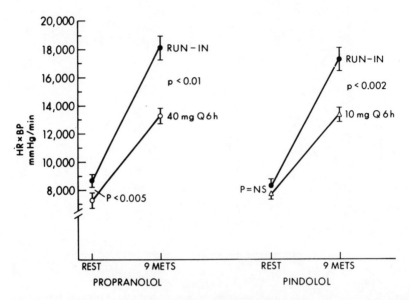

Figure 9-4. Effects of pindolol and propranolol on the HR × BP at rest and during exercise (9 mets). A significant decrease in resting HR × BP is seen with propranolol (160 mg per day) compared to the run-in period. The rate of increase in HR × BP during exercise was blunted with propranolol (160 mg per day) compared to the run-in period. A slight but insignificant decrease in resting HR × BP is seen with pindolol (40 mg per day) compared to the run-in period. The rate of increase in HR × BP during exercise is blunted with pindolol (40 mg per day) compared to the run-in period.

small but not significant decrease in the HR × BP was seen with pindolol, 8254 ±418 to 7651 ±210 mm Hg-min^{-1}!

Thus, pindolol did not appreciably change the resting heart rate, systolic blood pressure, or HR × BP, while a significant decrease in both resting heart rate and HR × BP was seen in patients treated with propranolol (Figs. 9-2-9-4, Table 9-1.). By analysis of variance, a more pronounced depression of heart rate was induced by propranolol than by pindolol.

EFFECTS OF PINDOLOL AND PROPRANOLOL ON EXERCISE TOLERANCE AND HR × BP

Exercise performance on the treadmill improved in both the propranolol and pindolol groups (Fig. 9-5). In the 23 patients receiving pindolol 10 mg every 6 hours the exercise capacity of patients improved from 8.0 ±0.4 to 9.7 ±0.3 mets ($p < 0.01$), while the exercise capacity of the 18 patients on propranolol, 40 mg every 6 hours, improved from 8.1 ±0.4 to 9.6 ±0.3 mets ($p < 0.05$). Similarly, the HR × BP at the end-

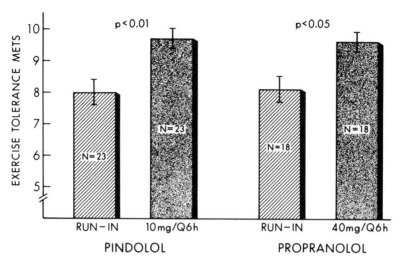

Figure 9-5. Effects of pindolol and propranolol on exercise tolerance in patients with angina pectoris. A significant improvement in mean total work performance occurs with both pindolol and propranolol compared to the run-in period.

point of exercise decreased from 17,540 ±827 to 15,276 ±736 mm Hg-min^{-1} with pindolol (p < 0.01); 17,182 ±1064 to 14,561 ±963 mm Hg-min^{-1} with propranolol (p < 0.001). Although all patients had developed angina at the end-point of exercise during the run-in phase, at peak dose none of the 23 patients on pindolol and 10 of the 18 patients on propranolol were forced to stop exercising because of fatigue and dsypnea rather than by angina.

Using analysis of variance there were no differences seen between pro-pranolol and pindolol with regards to β-blocker induced changes in exercise tolerance and decrements in HR × BP at exercise endpoint.

EFFECTS OF PINDOLOL AND PROPRANOLOL ON PATIENTS EXERCISING AT A GIVEN EXERCISE LEVEL (9 Mets)

When patients were exercising at the same level (9 mets), the magni-tude of the exercise-induced ECG ST-segment depression decreased from 1.3 ±0.3 mm during the run-in period to 0.4 ±0.15 mm in patients receiving pindolol (p < 0.05), and from 1.3 ±0.3 to 0.8 ±0.2 mm (p < 0.05) in pa-tients receiving propranolol (Fig. 9-6). Using analysis of variance, there was no difference between pindolol and propranolol in their effects on the exer-cise-induced ECG ST-segment depression.

At 9 mets, the heart rate of patients receiving pindolol decreased from

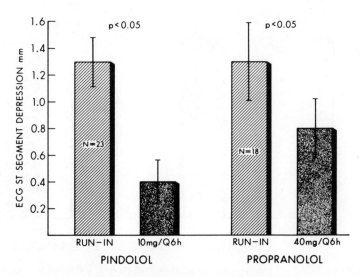

Figure 9-6. Effects of pindolol and propranolol on the ECG ST-segment at the 9 met exercise level. There is a significant reduction in the degree of ST segment depression in pindolol- and propranolol-treated patients compared to the run-in period.

114.2 ±4.1 (run-in) to 99.5 ±2.9 beats per minutes (pindolol 10 mg every 6 hours), $p < 0.002$. The heart rate of patients receiving propranolol decreased from 119.6 ±4.6 (run-in) to 95.7 ±2.3 beats per minute (propranolol 40 mg every 6 hours), $p < 0.004$. At 9 mets the systolic blood pressure decreased from 151.8 ±4.3 (run-in) to 132.7 ±2.3 mm Hg (pindolol 10 mg every 6 hours), $p < 0.01$, and from 152.2 ±6.2 (run-in) to 137.8 ±3.3 mm Hg in patients receiving propranolol (40 mg every 6 hours), $p < 0.05$ (Figs. 9-2, 9-3).

At the 9 met exercise level, the HR × BP decreased from 17,420 ±850 (run-in) to 13,205 ±510 mm Hg·min⁻¹ in patients receiving pindolol 10 mg every 6 hours, ($p < 0.002$). Similarly, the HR × BP decreased from 18,106 ±840 (run-in) to 13,255 ±480 mm Hg·min⁻¹ ($p < 0.01$) in patients receiving propranolol 40 mg every 6 hours (Fig. 9-4). There was no significant difference by analysis of variance between propranolol and pindolol on their effect on heart rate, blood pressure, and HR × BP at the 9 met exercise level.

WITHDRAWAL OF PINDOLOL AND PROPRANOLOL

An increase in the frequency of angina attacks occurred in both treatment groups during the 2-week withdrawal period. We did not observe death, myocardial infarction, or unstable angina requiring hospitalization in any patient, however.

ECHOCARDIOGRAPHIC MEASUREMENTS (Table 9-1)

The echocardiographically measured end-diastolic volume measured at rest showed an increase after pindolol (10 mg every 6 hours), from 70.8 ±1.8 (run-in) to 80.2 ±2.8 ml per m³, p < 0.02. A more pronounced increase in end-diastolic volume was seen in patients receiving propranolol (40 mg every 6 hours), from 71.8 ±3.2 (run-in) to 92.2 ±1.9 ml per m³, p < 0.003 (Fig. 9-7).

The echocardiographically estimated ejection fraction increased slightly in patients receiving pindolol (10 mg every 6 hours) compared to the run-in period, 0.59 ±0.02 to 0.62 ±0.02, p < 0.02. In contrast, propranolol (40 mg every 6 hours) decreased the ejection fraction from 0.57 ±0.02 (run-in) to 0.51 ±0.01, p < 0.04 (Fig. 9-8).

Using analysis of variance, the more pronounced increase in end-diastolic volume induced by propranolol as compared to pindolol was significant (p < 0.03). The differential effect of pindolol and propranolol on the resting ejection fraction was also significant (p < 0.002).

SIDE EFFECTS

The frequency and types of side effects seen with pindolol and propranolol treatment are listed in Table 9-2. Fatigue was a significant side ef-

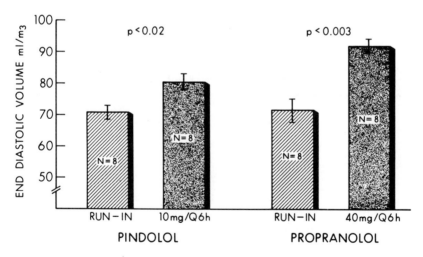

Figure 9-7. Effects of pindolol and propranolol on the left ventricular end-diastolic volume correction determined from the echocardiogram. Compared with the run-in period, there is a significant increase in end-diastolic volume with pindolol (40 mg per day) and propranolol (160 mg per day). The increase in end-diastolic volume with propranolol is significantly greater than that seen with pindolol.

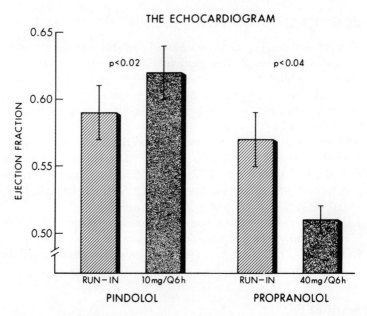

Figure 9-8.   Effects of pindolol and propranolol in the left ventricular ejection fraction determined from the echocardiogram. Compared with the run-in period, there is a slight but significant increase in the ejection fraction with pindolol (40 mg per day), and a decrease in this parameter with propranolol (160 mg per day). The effects of pindolol and propranolol on the ejection fraction are significantly different.

TABLE 9-2.   **Adverse Reactions**
Seen in Patients Treated with
Pindolol (N = 23) and Propranolol (N = 18)

Nature of Reaction	Number of Patients
Pindolol	
Nasal Stuffiness	1
Nocturia	1
Impotence	1
Palpitations	1
Total with adverse reactions	4
Propranolol	
Rash	1
Blurred vision	2
Fatigue	8
Dyspnea on exertion	1
Mild hypotension	5
Total with adverse reactions	17

fect seen in 1 out of 18 patients treated with propranolol. This adverse reaction was not seen in patients treated with pindolol.

DISCUSSION

β-Adrenoceptor blocking drugs are the greatest advance in the pharmacologic treatment of angina pectoris since the introduction of nitrates years ago. These agents work by reducing the heart rate, thus decreasing myocardial oxygen demands and allowing more time for diastolic coronary artery perfusion.[4,5] β-Blockade also reduces the sympathetically mediated rise in blood pressure with exercise, and the velocity of cardiac contraction.[1] Patients treated with these agents can do more exercise at a lower heart rate-blood pressure product (an indirect measure of myocardial oxygen consumption).[26]

Propranolol has proven effective in most patients with angina pectoris. The drug is a noncardioselective (affecting both β_1- and β_2-receptors) β-blocker with membrane depressant effects and lacks intrinsic sympathomimetic activity (ISA).[21] Propranolol is contraindicated in patients with active asthma and congestive heart failure since these conditions may be aggravated.[11]

Pindolol (LB-46) is a new β-adrenoceptor blocking drug with the most pronounced intrinsic sympathomimetic activity (partial agonist activity) of agents currently available.[12] Studies in reserpinized and adrenalectomized animals have shown that pindolol possesses this partial agonist effect unrelated to its β-blocking properties.[27] Pindolol is noncardioselective and has weaker membrane depressant activity than propranolol.[8,28] Unlike propranolol, it lacks "first-pass" metabolism.[21]

The drug has been shown, in multiple clinical trials, to be an effective antiarrhythmic[14,29,30] antihypertensive,[15,31] and antianginal agent.[16,32] Despite pindolol's proven clinical effectiveness, it has still not been determined whether intrinsic sympathomimetic activity is advantageous or disadvantageous in cardiac therapy. This partial agonist property has been claimed, by some investigators, to protect against myocardial failure,[17] however, comparative studies using compounds with (alprenolol) and without this property have revealed conflicting results.[33,34] It is known that compounds with ISA produce less depression of atrioventricular conduction[35] and smaller elevations of peripheral vascular resistance for a given degree of β-receptor blockade.[36] Similarly, agents lacking intrinsic sympathomimetic activity depress the resting heart rate more readily than those agents with ISA.[37]

Some clinical investigators have postulated that ISA would detract from β-blockade and, therefore, negate any therapeutic effectiveness in patients.[21,22] Our results show that pindolol and propranolol are equally effective in patients with angina pectoris when equipotent doses are used (pindolol 10 mg orally four times daily, propranolol 41 mg orally four times daily). Both drugs reduce the frequency of angina pectoris attacks and improve exercise tolerance. At a comparable exercise level (9 mets), there are similar effects for both drugs on the ECG ST-segment, systolic blood pressure, heart rate, and heart rate-blood pressure product when compared to the run-in period. Thus both pindolol and propranolol can improve exercise tolerance equally while at the same time reducing myocardial oxygen demands.

At rest, pindolol and propranolol had similar effects on the systolic blood pressure. Pindolol had no appreciable effect on resting heart rate, in contrast to propranolol, where a marked reduction in this parameter was noted. The rate-pressure product, though not significantly different with the two drugs, tended to be lower with propranolol (probably related to its greater rate-lowering effects).

An explanation for the similar effects of the drugs seen at exercise, and the differences at rest, probably relates to the intrinsic sympathomimetic activity of pindolol. ISA should be more pronounced at rest (a state of decreased sympathetic tone), and an increase in heart rate, secondary to this property, would counterbalance a decrease in rate caused by β-blockade. Thus, the resting heart rate would not change with pindolol (as shown in this study) whereas propranolol (lacking agonist activity) would decrease the resting heart rate. During exercise, however, where there is marked sympathetic stimulation, the β-blocking effects of pindolol would be more pronounced and markedly outweigh the direct stimulatory effects of intrinsic sympathomimetic activity, which is a factor dependent on dose and not underlying sympathetic tone. Thus, in states of high adrenergic activity, all β-adrenoceptor blocking drugs should be equally efficacious (whether or not they have intrinsic sympathomimetic activity), a fact that is born out by clinical trials demonstrating the clinical effectiveness of all β-blocking agents in exercise-induced angina pectoris.[10]

Pindolol was also shown, from echocardiographic studies done at rest, to be less of a myocardial depressant than propranolol. Pindolol was shown to cause a slight increase in the echocardiographically determined ejection fraction and end-diastolic volume. Propranolol caused a decrease in ejection fraction and a greater increment in end-diastolic volume.

The greater resting end-diastolic volume increment with propranolol may have been related to its rate-lowering effects and a greater time for diastolic filling. The maintenance of the resting ejection fraction with pindolol probably results from its stimulating ISA, counteracting the negative inotropic effects of β-adrenoceptor blockade in a low adrenergic state. In contrast, propranolol, lacking partial agonist activity, slightly depressed the ejection fraction at rest. Whether or not the effects on the ejection fraction would differ between propranolol and pindolol in the hyperadrenergic state seen with exercise has yet to be determined. One could speculate that the drugs in the setting of intense exercise and increased sympathetic tone would behave in a similar fashion (intrinsic sympathomimetic activity should no longer be important).

Recently, great attention has been directed towards the dangers of abrupt β-blocker withdrawal in patients with angina pectoris.[38,39] In this study, both pindolol and propranolol were safely withdrawn using the gradual regimen described in the methods section; all the patients in both treatment groups experienced a recrudescence of their angina pectoris symptomology when treatment was gradually withdrawn. No patient, however, developed unstable or crescendo angina requiring hospitalization, an acute myocardial infarction, or sudden death. Thus, β-adrenoceptor blocking drugs can be safely withdrawn after chronic therapy if done in a gradual fashion.

With regard to adverse reactions, pindolol is a relatively safe drug that differs from propranolol by causing less fatigue in patients. Whether this observation is related to the presence of ISA remains speculative.

Pindolol, with its intrinsic sympathomimetic activity, is an effective alternative to propranolol in patients with exercise-induced angina pectoris. Pindolol would appear to be advantageous for patients with resting sinus bradycardia where propranolol might be contraindicated. Pindolol might also be a safer β-adrenoceptor blocker in patients with angina pectoris and mild to moderate congestive heart failure. Pindolol can also be used where fatigue is a problem with propranolol. From studies done in patients with supraventricular arrhythmias and bronchospasm, it might also appear to be a better agent in patients with both angina pectoris and bronchial asthma.[20] On the other hand, pindolol does not lower the resting heart rate of patients. In patients who have angina pectoris at rest or at low exercise levels, therefore, propranolol would probably be more effective.

In conclusion, intrinsic sympathomimetic activity does not interfere with the therapeutic effectiveness of pindolol in exercising patients with angina pectoris. This property might also provide a protective effect in patients with unacceptable bradycardia or congestive heart failure at rest.

There are real differences between pindolol and propranolol which might be clinically useful, reinforcing the need to have multiple β-adrenoceptor blockings available to the practicing physician.

SUMMARY

Pindolol, a new β-adrenergic blocking drug with intrinsic sympathomimetic activity, and propranolol were given in increasing equipotent doses (pindolol: 2.5 to 10 mg every 6 hours; propranolol: 10 to 40 mg every 6 hours) over 12 weeks in a double-blind randomized trial to 41 patients with angina pectoris. The drugs were then gradually withdrawn over a 2-week period. With maximum doses, both pindolol and propranolol increased exercise capacity, compared to control, on multistage treadmill testing (pindolol: 8.0 +0.4 to 9.7 ±0.3 mets, p < 0.01; propranolol: 8.1 ±0.4 to 9.6 ±0.3 mets, p < 0.05). At each exercise level, both pindolol and propranolol decreased the heart rate, systolic blood pressure, and rate pressure product (HR × BP). At the 9 met exercise level, the HR × BP decreased from 17,420 ±850 to 13,205 ±510 mm Hg-min^{-1} with pindolol, (p < 0.002); with propranolol: 18,106 ±440 to 13,255 ±480 mm Hg-min^{-1} (p < 0.01). At the same level, the magnitude of exercise-induced ECG ST-depression decreased from 1.3 ±0.3 to 0.4 ±0.15 mm with pindolol (p < 0.05) and from 1.3 ±0.3 to 0.8 ±0.2 mm with propranolol (p < 0.05). Both drugs reduced the number of spontaneous attacks of angina pectoris per week. Pindolol did not appreciably decrease the resting heart rate (66.8 ±1.9 versus 64.6 ±1.2) or HR × BP (8254 ±418 versus 7651 ±210 mm Hg-min^{-1}) in contrast to propranolol which reduced both (heart rate: 70.5 ±2.2 to 62.2 ±2.4, p < 0.01; HR × BP: 8677 ±423 to 7338 ±455 mm Hg-min^{-1}, p < 0.005). In addition, pindolol slightly decreased the echocardiographically estimated ejection fraction at rest (0.59 ±0.02 to 0.62 ±0.02, p < 0.02), while propranolol depressed it (0.57 ±0.02 to 0.51 ±0.01, p < 0.04). Both pindolol and propranolol could be safely withdrawn over a gradual 2-week withdrawal interval.

CONCLUSIONS

1. Both pindolol and propranolol are effective in the symptomatic relief of angina pectoris.
2. Pindolol is preferable in patients with resting bradycardia or congestive heart failure, while propranolol may be more effective in patients with angina at rest or at very low exercise levels.
3. The two drugs can be safely withdrawn if done in a gradual fashion.
4. Intrinsic sympathomimetic activity does not interfere with the therapeutic benefit of β-blockade in angina pectoris.

REFERENCES

1. Sowton E, Humor J: Hemodynamic changes after beta-adrenergic blockade. Am J Cardiol 18: 317–320, 1966
2. Robinson BF: The mode of action of beta-antagonists in angina pectoris. Postgrad Med J 47 (Suppl 2): 41–43, 1971

3. Robinson BF: Relation of heart rate and systolic pressure to the onset of pain in angina pectoris. Circulation 35: 1073-1083, 1967

4. Thadani U, Sharma B, Meeran MK, et al.: Comparison of adrenergic beta-receptor antagonists in angina pectoris. Br Med J 1: 138-142, 1973

5. Wolfson S, Gorlin R: Cardiovascular pharmacology of propranolol in man. Circulation 40: 501-511, 1969

6. Frishman WH, Weksler B, Christodoulou J, Smithen C, Killip T: Reversal of abnormal platelet aggregability and change in exercise tolerance in patients with angina pectoris following oral propranolol. Circulation 50: 887-896, 1974

7. Frishman WH, Smithen C, Christodoulou J, et al.: Medical management of angina pectoris: multifactoral action of propranolol. In Norman J, Cooley D (eds): Coronary Artery Medicine and Surgery. New York, Appleton, 1975, pp 285-294

8. Frishman WH: Clinical pharmacology of the new beta adrenergic blocking drugs. Part 1: Pharmacodynamic and pharmacokinetic properties. Am Heart J 97: 663-670, 1979

9. Frishman WH, Silverman R: Clinical pharmacology of the new beta adrenergic blocking drugs. Part 2: Physiologic and metabolic effects. Am Heart J 97: 797-807, 1979

10. Frishman WH, Silverman R: Clinical pharmacology of the new beta adrenergic blocking drugs. Part 3: Comparative clinical experience and new therapeutic applications. Am Heart J 98: 119-131, 1979

11. Frishman WH, Silverman R, Strom J, et al.: Clinical pharmacology of the new beta adrenergic blocking drugs. Part 4: adverse effects. Choosing a β-adrenoreceptor blocker. Am Heart J 98: 256-262, 1979

12. Barrett AM, Carter J: Comparative chronotropic activity of β-adrenoceptive antagonists. Br J Pharmacol 40: 373-381, 1970

13. Levi GF, Proto C: Combined treatment of atrial fibrillation with quinidine and beta-blockers. Br Heart J 34: 911-914, 1972

14. Aronow WS, Uyeyama RR: Treatment of arrhythmias with pindolol. Clin Pharmacol Ther 13: 15-22, 1972

15. Simpson FO, Waal-Manning HI: Comparison of pindolol (Visken) with other antihypertensive drugs. Aust NZ J Med 3: 425-426, 1973

16. Sainani GS, Mukherjee AK: A double-blind of LB-46 (Visken) in angina pectoris. Ind Heart J 24 (Suppl. 1): 192-196, 1972

17. Ablad B, Brogard M, Ek L: Pharmacological properties of H56/28 — a beta-adrenergic receptor antagonist. Acta Pharmacol Fox 25 (Suppl 2): 9, 1967

18. Gugler R, Hobel W, Badem G, Dengler HJ: The effect of pindolol on exercise-induced cardiac acceleration in relation to plasma levels in man. Clin Pharmacol Ther 17: 127-133, 1975

19. Beumer HM, Hardonk HJ: Effects of beta-adrenergic blocking drugs on ventilatory function in asthmatics. Eur J Clin Pharmacol 5: 77-80, 1972

20. Frishman WH, Davis R, Strom J, et al.: Clinical Pharmacology of the New Beta Adrenergic Blocking Drugs. Part 5: Pindolol (LB-46) therapy for supraventricular arrhythmia: a viable alternative to propranolol in patients with bronchospasm. Am Heart J 98: 393-398, 1979

21. Conolly ME, Kersting F, Dollery CT: The clinical pharmacology of beta-adrenoceptor blocking drugs. Prog Cardiovasc Dis 19: 203-234, 1976

22. Turner P: β-adrenergic receptor blocking drugs in hyperthyroidism. Drugs 7: 48-54, 1974

23. Popp RL, Alderman EL, Brown OR, Harrison DC: Sources of error in calculation of left ventricular volume by echocardiography (abstr.). Am J Cardiol 31: 152, 1973
24. Fortuin NJ, Hood WP, Craige E: Evaluation of left ventricular volume by echocardiography. Circulation 46: 26-35, 1972
25. Pombo JF, Troy BL, Russell RO: Left ventricular volume and ejection fraction by echocardiography. Circulation 43: 480-490, 1971
26. Frishman W, Smithen C, Befler B, Kligfield P, Killip T: Non-invasive assessment of clinical response to oral propranolol therapy. Am J Cardiol 35: 635-644, 1975
27. Barrett AM, Nunn B: Intrinsic sympathomimetic activity in relation to the precipitation of heart failure by beta adrenoceptive blockade. Arch Int Pharmacodyn Ther 189: 168-174, 1971
28. Levy JV: Cardiovascular effects of pindolol (LB-46), a potent beta-adrenergic receptor antagonist. J Clin Pharmacol 11: 249-260, 1971
29. Storstein L: LB-46, a new beta-adrenergic receptor blocking agent in cardiac arrhythmias. Acta Med Scand 191: 423-428, 1972
30. Kimura E: Some clinical aspects of the effects of beta-blocking agents especially LB-46. New Horizons Med 1: 85-88, 1970
31. Feltham PM, Watson OF, Peel JS, Dunlop OJ, Turner AS: Pindolol in hypertension: a double-blind trial. NZ Med J 76: 161-171, 1972
32. Nair DV: A double-blind trial of Visken 1 LB-46, in the treatment of angina pectoris. Ind Heart J 3 (Suppl 1): 183-191, 1972
33. Lund-Larsen PG, Silvertssen E: Hemodynamic effects of propranolol (inderal) and H56/28 Aptin in patients with acute myocardial infarction. A comparative study. Acta Med Scand 186: 187-191, 1969
34. Wasserman AJ, Proctor JD, Allen FJ, Kemp VE: Human cardiovascular effects of alprenolol, a beta-adrenergic blocker; hemodynamic, anti-arrhythmic, and anti-anginal. J Clin Pharmacol 10: 37-49, 1970
35. Morgan TO, Sabto J, Anavekar SM, Louis WJ, Doyle AE: A comparison of beta adrenergic blocking drugs in the treatment of hypertension. Postgrad Med J 50: 253-259, 1974
36. Imhof PR: Characterization of beta blockers as anti-hypertensive agents in the light of human pharmacology. In Schweizer W (ed): Beta-Blockers — Present Status and Future Prospects. Bern, Huber, 1974, pp 40-50
37. Prichard BNC, Aellig WH, Richardson GA: The action of intravenous oxprenolol, practolol, propranolol, and sotalol on acute exercise tolerance in angina pectoris: The effect on heart rate and the electrocardiogram. Postgrad Med J 46 (Nov Suppl): 77-85, 1970
38. Miller RR, Olson HG, Amsterdam EA, Mason DT: Propranolol withdrawal rebound phenomenon: exacerbation of coronary events after abrupt cessation of anti-anginal therapy. N Engl J Med 293: 416-418, 1975
39. Frishman WH, Christodoulou J, Weksler B, et al.: Abrupt propranolol withdrawal in angina pectoris: effects on platelet aggregation and exercise tolerance. Am Heart J 95: 169-179, 1978

CHAPTER TEN

Nadolol: A Long Acting Beta-Adrenoceptor Blocking Drug

William H. Frishman

T HE value of β-adrenergic blockade in arterial hypertension, angina pectoris, and arrhythmias has been well established during the last decade.[1] An increasing number of β-blockers with varying pharmacodynamic and pharmacokinetic properties have recently been introduced into clinical practice.[2]

Nadolol (SQ 11,275) is a new noncardioselective β-adrenergic blocking agent which was developed in the United States. It has a unique pharmacologic property in that it has the longest plasma half-life of any known β-blocking drug, and can be administered once daily.[3]

The clinical experience with nadolol is now being gathered world-wide in angina pectoris, arrhythmias, and hypertension. The first clinical trials in the United States have been completed using nadolol for the treatment of hypertension and angina pectoris and the drug has received FDA approval for these indications. In this chapter, the clinical pharmacology, efficacy, and toxicity of this promising new agent will be described, and its potential therapeutic applications discussed.

PHARMACODYNAMIC AND PHARMACOKINETIC PROPERTIES (Table 10-1)

Nadolol, 2,3-cis-1,2,3,4-tetrahydro-5- [2-hydroxy-3-tert-butylamine] propoxy -2,3, naphthalenediol (Fig. 10-1), is a nonselective β-adrenoceptor blocking drug which lacks both membrane-stabilizing and intrinsic sympathomimetic activity (partial agonist activity).[3,4] It has a level of potency which is 2 to 4 times that of propranolol.[3] Compared to propranolol, nadolol (probably related to its lack of membrane-stabilizing effect) has been found to be approximately 50 to 500 times less depressant to the isolated guinea pig atrium.[5]

TABLE 10-1. A Comparison Between the Pharmacologic Properties of Propranolol and Nadolol

Pharmacologic Property	Propranolol	Nadolol
β-blockade potency ratio (propranolol = 1)	1	2-4
Cardioselectivity	0	0
Partial agonist activity	0	0
Membrane-stabilizing activity	+	0
Extent of absorption (% of oral dose)	>90	≅30
First pass hepatic metabolism	+	0
Protein binding (%)	≅90	≅30
Elimination half-life (hours)	3.5-6	17-24
Urinary and fecal recovery of unchanged drug (% of oral dose)	<1	<90
Active metabolites	+	0

Nadolol is absorbed rapidly from the gastrointestinal tract achieving its peak effect in 3 to 4 hours.[6] Only 30 percent of the oral dose is absorbed.[6,7] The drug is not metabolized in the body and is excreted unchanged in the urine (70 percent of absorbed dose) and via the bile in the feces (20 percent of absorbed dose).[6-8] Nadolol is 30 percent bound to plasma proteins.[7] The drug has a plasma half-life of 17 to 23 hours, the longest of any known β-blocker.[6,7] The plasma half-life is even longer where there is renal dysfunction, with elimination proportional to creatine clearance. The drug can be removed with hemodialysis.

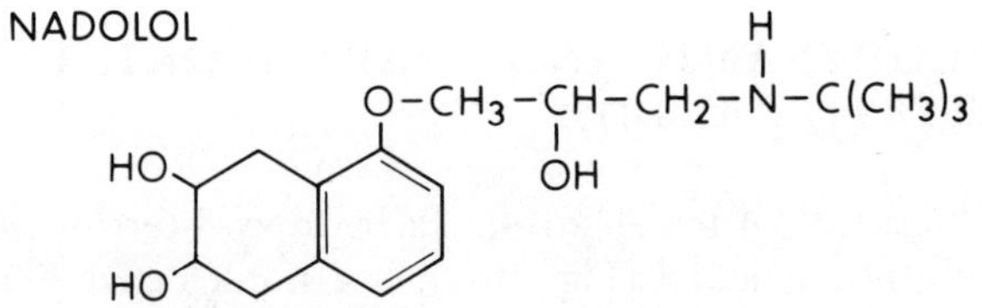

NADOLOL

$$O-CH_3-CH-CH_2-\overset{\overset{\textstyle H}{\textstyle |}}{N}-C(CH_3)_3$$

Figure 10-1. Structural formula of the β-adrenoceptor blocking drug, nadolol.

PHYSIOLOGIC AND METABOLIC EFFECTS (Table 10-2)

The hemodynamic effects of nadolol are attributable to β-adrenoceptor blockade. In human studies, nadolol, like propranolol, reduces cardiac contractility and work. In a hemodynamic study of 14 patients with coronary artery disease, both nadolol and propranolol (in similar β-blocking doses) reduced heart rate, cardiac index, stroke work, ejection fraction, dp/dt, and V_{MAX}; peripheral resistance rose slightly.[9] The cardiocirculatory effects of nadolol and propranolol were similar. In another study employing radionucleotide techniques to evaluate left ventricular function in patients with coronary artery disease, both nadolol and propranolol (in equivalent β-blocking concentrations) reduced the ejection fraction.[10]

TABLE 10-2.   Hemodynamic and Electrophysiologic Effects
of Propranolol and Nadolol*

Hemodynamic Parameter	Propranolol	Nadolol
Resting heart rate	↓	↓
Exercise induced increment in heart rate	↓	↓
Peripheral resistance	↔↑	↔↑
Effect on blood pressure (rest)	↓	↓
Exercise induced increment in blood pressure	↓	↓
Cardiac contractility	↓	↓↔
Cardiac output	↓	↓
Effect on elevated plasma renin	↓	↓
Effect on atrioventricular conduction	↓	↓

*In dosages giving similar degree of β-blockade.

The findings of the above studies differ from the results of animal experiments where nadolol was found to have less myocardial depressant effect than propranolol. These experiments were done in the isolated guinea pig atria and the membrane-stabilizing action of propranolol may have been important with the concentrations of drug used.[3]

In several experimental studies, nadolol has been demonstrated to be effective against cardiac arrhythmias.[4,11-14] As seen with other β-blocking agents, this antiarrhythmic activity appears to be related to β-adrenergic receptor blockade, an action that would antagonize the ability of catecholamines to induce arrhythmias by alteration of cardiac automaticity and conductivity.[4,12-14]

Nadolol was effective in antagonizing ectopic activity occurring during vagal-induced depression of primary pacemaker activity, presumably by inhibiting the actions of catecholamines on the automaticity of the ectopic pacemaker. Both nadolol and propranolol antagonized isoproterenol-induced tachycardia, and oubain-induced arrhythmias, in cats. The two agents also antagonized coronary-artery-ligation-induced ventricular fibrillation. In contrast to propranolol, nadolol was considerably weaker in suppressing existing digoxin-induced arrhythmias and lacked membrane-stabilizing activity. Both nadolol and propranolol depress atrioventricular conduction.[4] The duration of β-blocker effect was five times greater with nadolol than with propranolol.[4]

Nadolol has been shown to have similar effects on glucose and lipid metabolism as propranolol.[15] With regard to other physiologic parameters (effects on the bronchial tree, platelet function, hemoglobin-oxygen dissociation), there are insufficient data.

Nadolol has been shown, both in animal experiments and human trials, to lower pretreatment plasma renin activity as much as 50 percent.[7,16] This decrease in plasma renin activity is in the same range as earlier reported for hypertensive patients treated with propranolol. In preliminary studies (animal and human), nadolol has been shown to increase renal blood flow. This finding contrasts with the observations made with all other β-blocking drugs where renal blood flow has been shown to decrease due to decreased cardiac output. The mechanism for this paradoxical renal blood flow effect with nadolol has not been elucidated.

THERAPEUTIC APPLICATIONS AND CLINICAL EXPERIENCE

The hemodynamic and pharmacokinetic profile of action of nadolol suggested its application in cardiovascular disorders such as hypertension,[1,16] ischemic heart disease, and cardiac arrhythmias.

HYPERTENSION

It is well recognized that β-adrenergic blocking agents are effective in controlling the blood pressure of many patients with hypertension.[1,17] As mentioned previously, there is no consensus of opinion as to the mechanism, or mechanisms, by which these drugs lower blood pressure. Moreover, there appears to be no difference in therapeutic efficacy between the different β-blockers (with a similar degree of β-blockade) in hypertension.[1,17]

Nadolol has proven to be a safe and effective antihypertensive agent when compared with placebo. A preliminary, single-blind study was carried out with nadolol in 30 untreated patients with essential hypertension.[16] After a 2-week period on placebo, patients were treated for 14 weeks, commencing with daily doses of 40 mg nadolol (20 mg twice daily). Dosage was increased every second week up to a maximum of 560 mg daily until the patient was stabilized at an effective normotensive dose level. Compared to placebo, there was a significant reduction in both systolic and diastolic blood pressure (approximately 24/21 mm Hg) at an average daily dose of 110 mg nadolol. Pretreatment plasma renin activity value decreased by 50 percent as a result of 14 weeks treatment with nadolol. This decrease in plasma renin activity is in the same range as earlier reported for hypertensive patients treated with propranolol. Apart from a tendency to bradycardia, no other side effects were reported.

The long half-life of nadolol in serum suggested the possibility of administering the drug only once a day. Many trials are currently in progress comparing the efficacy of oral nadolol, administered once daily, with propranolol administered four times daily.

A drug which can be taken once daily could enhance patient compliance in treatment of hypertension. Studies have shown that patient compliance in hypertension varies with the complexity of the dosing regimens.[18,19] In one large study of a hypertensive population, only 5 percent of patients given a diuretic failed to take the prescribed dose presumably due to the simplicity of the once-a-day therapeutic regimen, whereas, the proportion not taking α-methyldopa, propranolol, and reserpine (multiple dose regimen) approached 31 percent.[18] This lack of patient compliance was unrelated to side effects.

Would a β-blocking drug with a 24-hour half-life, therefore, be an advantage in therapy of hypertension? Propranolol and oxprenolol have comparatively short half-lives, and if this alone determined the frequency of drug dosage, these agents would need to be given at least four times daily.[2] However, the physiologic effect of β-blockade upon blood pressure substantially outlasts the survival of unchanged drug in the plasma: twice or even once daily dosage seems adequate.[2,20,21] Therefore, preparations with a long pharmacokinetic half-life such as nadolol and atenolol, or slow-release preparations of drugs such as oxprenolol, may confer no great advantage.

ANGINA PECTORIS

Multiple studies have demonstrated the effectiveness of β-adrenoceptor blocking agents for the treatment of patients with angina pectoris. As described previously, these drugs reduce the determinants of myocardial oxygen consumption enabling a patient to do more work.[2,17]

A randomized, double-blind study was carried out in 24 patients with stable angina pectoris to compare the efficacy of nadolol and propranolol.[22] After a period on placebo, 14 patients received nadolol once daily and 10 patients, propranolol four times daily, over a 10-week dose ranging period, followed by a maintenance period of 4 weeks. The optimal daily dosage for nadolol was 100 mg, and 112 mg for propranolol. The parameters used for evaluation of therapeutic effectiveness included the number of anginal attacks, number of nitroglycerin tablets needed, time before onset of chest pain during an exercise test, exercise time, and overall clinical impression. Nadolol and propranolol were equally effective in reducing anginal attacks and nitroglycerin consumption. Similarly, exercise tolerance was improved with both drugs.

It was concluded from this study that nadolol, once a day, is as effective as propranolol, four times daily, in treating patients with angina pectoris.

A β-blocker that can be given as a single daily dose for angina pectoris might be a factor of major importance in ensuring patient compliance. It is not known at this time, however, whether other β-blockers, with shorter half-lives, can also be given once or twice daily for angina pectoris.

A larger multicenter trial in this country comparing nadolol once daily with placebo and propranolol taken four times daily has been completed. The published results are being awaited with great interest.

ARRHYTHMIAS

Nadolol was initially developed as an antiarrhythmic agent in 1973.[4,11] As with all β-adrenoceptor blocking drugs, its antiarrhythmic properties stem from the ability to antagonize the effects of catecholamines on cardiac automaticity and conductivity.[1] Although the electrophysiologic properties of the drug are well known, there is no large clinical data base to date.

In one study, 29 patients with frequent ventricular and supraventricular ectopic beats and other supraventricular arrhythmias, received sequential doses of placebo and nadolol.[14] Dose titration and nadolol maintenance were accomplished during a four week period on doses up to 100 mg per day, preceded and followed by placebo periods extending to 2 weeks. Ectopic activity was monitored by Holter 24-hour dynamic electrocardiography. A reduction of remission of arrhythmia was observed in approximately two-thirds of patients. Arrhythmias that responded favorably involved ventricular bigeminy, paroxysmal atrial tachycardia, and sinus tachycardia. Patients with atrial flutter or fibrillation did not convert to normal sinus rhythm, however, all patients had a favorable reduction in ventricular response. Maintenance doses most frequently used were 60 to 160 mg per day, in single or divided doses. Reductions in resting heart rate and arterial pressure, consistent with β-adrenoceptor blockade, were observed. It was concluded from this trial that nadolol might be of value in the treatment of cardiac dysrhythmias.

A β-blocker with a long half-life, administered once daily for management of cardiac arrhythmias, might prove extremely useful in clinical practice. Comparisons with other β-blockers and other antiarrhythmic agents are still necessary for evaluating the usefulness of nadolol, once a day, in the acute and chronic treatment of patients with cardiac dysrhythmias.

SIDE EFFECTS AND TOXICITY

In the limited clinical experience to date, nadolol has side effects similar to other β-adrenoceptor blocking drugs (i.e., propranolol).[14,16,22] No unusual toxic effects have been demonstrated and carcinogenicity study requirements have been met.[23]

One potential problem with chronic nadolol administration might be the toxic accumulation of the drug in the plasma of patients with impaired renal function. With its long half-life, lack of hepatic metabolism, and renal elimination property, nadolol dosage must be varied according to the serum creatinine.[6] In situations where toxic levels of the drug might accumulate, the drug is dialyzable.

THERAPEUTIC IMPLICATIONS AND CONCLUSIONS

Nadolol is an effective β-adrenoceptor blocking agent with the longest half-life among the compounds of this class. This property would enable the drug to be administered once daily and clinical studies have substantiated the effectiveness of this regimen. With the common problem of daily patient compliance in hypertension, arrhythmia, and angina pectoris, where multidose regimens are used, an agent which can be taken once daily would provide a major advantage. On the other hand, recent studies have suggested that the β-adrenoceptor blocking drugs with short half-lives have longer pharmacodynamic actions, which might obviate the need for their frequent dosing. Until this crucial pharmacologic issue is resolved, nadolol appears to be an important pharmacologic advance.

REFERENCES

1. Frishman W, Silverman R: Clinical pharmacology of the new beta-adrenergic blocking drugs. Part 2. Physiologic and metabolic effects. Am Heart J 97: 797, 1979
2. Frishman W: Clinical pharmacology of the new beta-adrenergic blocking drugs. Part 1. Pharmacodynamic and pharmacokinetic properties. Am Heart J 97: 663, 1979
3. Lee RJ, Evans DB, Baky SH, Laffa RJ: Pharmacology of nadolol (SQ 11,725), a beta-adrenergic antagonist lacking direct myocardial depression. Eur J Pharmacol 33: 371–382, 1975
4. Evans DB, Peschka MT, Lee RJ, Laffan RJ: Anti-arrhythmic action of nadolol, a beta-adrenergic receptor blocking compound. Eur J Pharmacol 35: 17–27, 1976

5. Lee RJ, Evans DB, Baky SH, Laffan RJ: The cardiovascular pharmacology of SQ 11,725 (SQ), a potent beta-adrenergic antagonist lacking significant myocardial depressant activity. Fed Proc 32: 780, 1973 (Abs)

6. Dreyfuss J, Brannick LJ, Vukovich RA, Shaw JM, Willard DA: Metabolic studies in patients with nadolol: oral and intravenous administration. J Clin Pharmacol 17: 300–307, 1977

7. Vukovich RA, Dreyfuss J, Brannick LJ, Herrera J, Willard DA: Pharmacologic and metabolic studies with a new beta-adrenergic blocking agent, nadolol. Clin Res 24: 52, 1976

8. Wong KK, Dreyfuss J, Shaw JM, Ross JJ Jr., Schreiber EC: A beta-blocking agent (SQ 11,725) that is not metabolized extensively by dogs and monkeys. Pharmacologist 15: 245, 1973 (Abs)

9. Lee G, DeMaria AN, Miller RR, et al.: Comparative effects of nadolol and propranolol on cardiac and peripheral circulatory function in patients with coronary artery disease. Clin Res 26:(2): 100A, 1978

10. LeWinter MM, Curtis G, Shabetai R, et al.: Comparison of the effects of a new beta-adrenergic blocking agent (nadolol) and propranolol on left ventricular performance in patients with prior myocardial infarction. Clin Res 26 (2): 101A, 1978

11. Peschka M, Evans DB, Laffan RJ: Anti-arrhythmic activity of SQ 11,725 (SQ), a potent nondepressant beta-adrenergic blocking agent. Fed Proc 32: 780, 1973 (Abs)

12. Gibson JK, Gelband H, Bassett AL: Possible basis of antiarrhythmic action of a new beta-adrenergic blocking compound. Am J Cardiol 37: 138, 1976 (Abs)

13. Gibson JK, Gelband H, Bassett AL: Effects of SQ 11,725 on the electrophysiology of isolated mitral cardiac tissue. Pharmacologist 16: 201, 1974 (Abs)

14. Vukovich RA, Sasahara A, Zombrano P, et al.: Antiarrhythmic effects of a new beta-adrenergic blocking agent, nadolol. Clin Pharmacol Ther 19: 118, 1976

15. McKinstry DN, Vukovich RA, Willard DA: Effects of beta-adrenergic blockade with nadolol and propranolol on glucose and lipid metabolism in man. Clin Res 25 (3): 548A, 1977

16. Frithz G: Dose-ranging study of the new beta-adrenergic antagonist nadolol in the treatment of essential hypertension. Curr Med Res Opin 5: 383, 1978

17. Frishman W, Silverman R: Clinical pharmacology of the new beta-adrenergic blocking drugs. Part 3. Comparative clinical experience and new therapeutic applications. Am Heart J 98: 119, 1979

18. Bulpitt CJ, Dollery CT: Side effects of hypotensive agents evaluated by a self-administered questionnaire. Br Med J 3: 485–490, 1973

19. Caldwell JR, Cobb S, Dowling MD, DeJongh D: The drop-out problem in antihypertensive treatment. J Chron Dis 22: 579

20. Berglund G, Anderson O, Hansson L, Olander R: Propranolol given twice daily in hypertension. Acta Med Scand 194: 513–515, 1973

21. Wilson M, Morgan G, Morgan T: The effect of blood pressure of β-adrenoreceptor-blocking drugs given once daily. Clin Sci Mole Med 51: 527s–528s, 1976

22. Furberg B, Dahlqvist A, Raak A, Wrege U: Comparison of the new beta-adrenoceptor antagonist, nadolol, and propranolol in the treatment of angina pectoris. Curr Med Res Opin 5: 388, 1978

23. Status report on beta blockers, FDA Drug Bulletin 8: 13, 1978

CHAPTER ELEVEN

New Horizons in Beta-Adrenoceptor Blocking Therapy: Labetalol

William H. Frishman

AHLQUIST has proposed that adrenoceptors consist of two distinct types, which he termed alpha (α) and beta (β), and there is overwhelming experimental and clinical evidence in support of this concept. Agonists, acting at one or both types of adrenoceptor, have been available for years. The situation with antagonists is different, however. Until recently, only antagonists acting at α- or β-adrenoceptors, but not at both, were available. Phentolamine is a typical α-adrenoceptor antagonist and propranolol, a typical β-adrenoceptor antagonist. In 1972, the pharmacology of a unique agent was described, labetalol, which had antagonist properties at both α-and β-adrenoreceptors.[2-4] Labetalol has recently been approved for use in hypertension in Great Britain and represents the forerunner of a new pharmacologic group of compounds with combined α- and β-adrenoceptor blocking properties.

The clinical experience with labetalol is now being gathered worldwide in angina pectoris, hypertension, and arrhythmias, with the first clinical trials beginning in the United States. In this chapter, the clinical pharmacology, efficacy, and toxicity of this promising new α-β-adrenoceptor blocking agent will be described, and its potential therapeutic applications discussed.

PHARMACODYNAMIC AND PHARMACOKINETIC PROPERTIES (Table 11-1)

PHARMACODYNAMIC PROPERTIES

Labetolol 5-(1-hydroxy-2-[(1 methyl-3 phenylpropyl) amino] ethyl) salicylamide (Fig. 11-1) is a competitive antagonist at both α- and β-adrenoceptors. Over the range of in vitro and in vivo tests used, labetalol has been shown to be 6 to 10 times less potent than phentolamine at α-adrenoceptors, 1.5 to 4 times less potent than propranolol at β-adrenoceptors, and was itself 4 to 16 times less potent at α- than at β-adrenoceptors.[5] Labetalol blocked α- and β-adrenoceptor-mediated sympathetic nerve stimulation to approximately the same extent as with exogenously administered phenylephrine or isoproterenol.[5]

TABLE 11-1. A Comparison Between the Pharmacologic Properties of Propranolol and Labetalol

Pharmacologic Property	Propranolol	Labetalol
β-blockade potency ratio (labetalol = 1)	1.5–4	1
α-adrenoceptor blocking effect	0	+
Cardioselectivity	0	0
Partial agonist activity	0	0
Membrane-stabilizing activity	+	+
Extent of absorption (% of oral dose)	>90	>90
First pass hepatic metabolism	+	+
Dose-dependent bioavailability	+	+
Lipid solubility	Strong	Weak
Active metabolites	+	−

The β-adrenoceptor-blocking action of labetalol, like propranolol, is nonselective.[5,6] It might therefore be expected that the drug would cause bronchoconstriction in asthmatics, as does propranolol.[6] In animal studies, labetalol has been shown to be 4 times less potent than propranolol in the heart, but about 11 times less potent on the lung.[5] If this applies clinically to patients with bronchial asthma, then at equipotent doses labetalol should cause less bronchoconstriction than propranolol. The α-adrenoceptor-blocking activity of labetalol might also be beneficial in asthmatics, since there is evidence that α-adrenoceptors are present in bronchial muscle and that their activation causes bronchoconstriction.[7,8] In man, α-adrenoceptor antagonists may have a bronchodilator action of their own, and have been shown to enhance the bronchodilator actions of isoproterenol and salbutamol.[9,10]

In view of the ability of labetalol to block both types of adrenoceptor, it was particularly important to resolve the question of its specificity. The blocking action of labetalol, both in vivo and in vitro, has been shown to be specific for α- and β-adrenoceptors. The drug has no antihistamine activity; however, there is recent evidence to suggest that it may have a direct vasodilator component. Vasodilators, such as diazoxide, characteristically reduce contractile responses of vascular muscle to a variety of spasmogens, whereas labetalol reduces contractile responses to norepinephrine only.[5]

Although labetalol is devoid of blocking actions at receptors other than adrenoceptors, it does possess additional actions. It has a direct negative inotropic action (unrelated to adrenoceptor blockade) which is probably a manifestation of membrane-stabilizing activity, a property shared by other β-adrenoceptor antagonists (including propranolol).[5] As with propranolol,[11] however, the direct negative inotropic effect (membrane-stabilizing property) of labetalol is unlikely to be clinically important, as this effect is apparent only at doses considerably higher than those required for α-or β-adrenoceptor blockade.[5]

In experiments with dogs, labetalol has been known not to possess agonist (intrinsic sympathomimetic) activity at cardiac β_1-adrenoceptors.[2]

PHARMACOKINETIC PROPERTIES (Table 11-1)

The absorption, distribution, and metabolism of labetalol has been studied in the rat, rabbit, dog, and man, as part of the pharmacologic, toxicologic, and clinical evaluation of the drug.

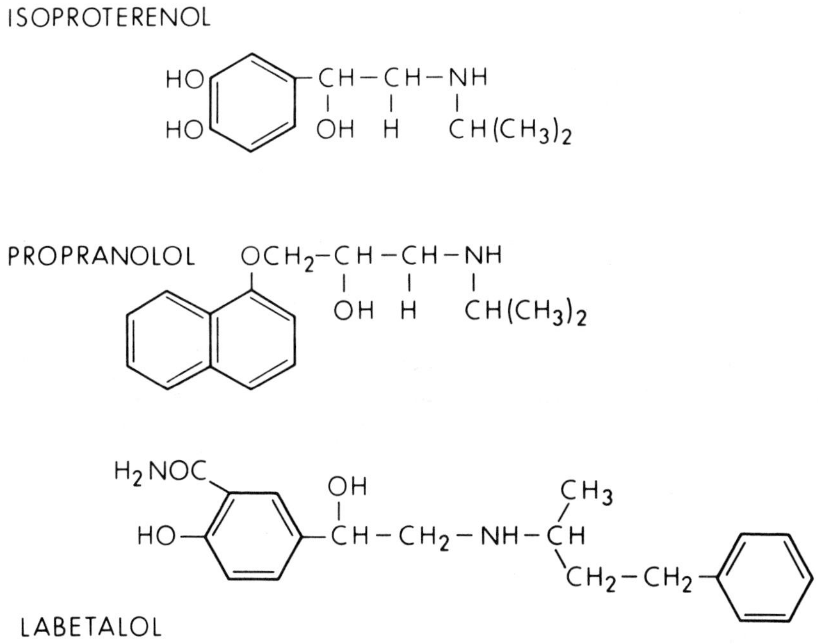

Figure 11-1. Structural formulas of the β-antagonist isoproterenol, the β-antagonist propranolol, and the α-β antagonist labetalol.

The plasma levels of radioactively labeled labetalol and high urinary excretion of radioactivity show that labetalol is well absorbed by man. The drug has a "first-pass" metabolism similar to that of propranolol so there may be a variation in bioavailability dependent on the dosage of drug administered.[12] The drug is quickly taken up by the tissues and rapidly cleared from the body via both kidneys and the bile.[12] Labetalol is much less lipophilic than other β-adrenoceptor blocking agents and, because of this, there is negligible uptake of labetalol in the brain.[12] However, there is a reversible binding of the drug to the melanin of the uveal tract in the eye.[12, 13]

Labetalol is metabolized in the liver by conjugation and the metabolites excreted by the kidney (50 percent) and via the bile into the feces (50 percent).[12] There is decreased metabolism of the drug in patients with hepatic disease, necessitating lower dosage. The pharmacokinetics of labetalol are being studied in patients with poor renal function.

Peak serum levels of the drug are seen 1 hour after oral administration. The therapeutic blood level of drug has been found to be 5 μg per ml in man.[12]

PHYSIOLOGIC AND METABOLIC EFFECTS (Table 11-2)

Labetalol has α- and β-adrenoceptor blocking properties both in man and animals. There have been some differences of opinion among investigators concerning physiologic effects of labetalol because it has a variety of properties, and the balance between those properties may change at different dose levels. It may be that at low doses of labetalol β-adrenoceptor-blocking properties predominate, whereas at higher doses α-adrenoceptor blocking properties are the most significant. The data concerning dose variable effects have not been obtained.

The hemodynamic effects of labetalol are attributable to its adreno-

TABLE 11-2.   Hemodynamic Effects of Propranolol and Labetalol*

Hemodynamic Parameter	Propranolol	Labetalol
Resting heart rate	↓↓	↓↔
Exercise induced increment in heart rate	↓	↓
Peripheral resistance	↔↑	↓
Effect on blood pressure (rest)	↓	↓↓
Exercise induced increment in blood pressure	↓	↓↓
Cardiac contractility	↓	↓↔
Cardiac output	↓	↔↓
Effect on elevated plasma renin	↓	↓

*In dosages giving similar degree of β-blockade.

ceptor-blocking actions.[5] In animal and human studies, labetalol, like propranolol, reduced cardiac contractility and work, effects attributable to β-adrenoceptor blockade.[5] Labetalol differed from propranolol in decreasing rather than increasing total peripheral resistance, and in causing larger falls in resting blood pressure at equipotent β-adrenoceptor blocking doses.[5] It seems reasonable to attribute these differences to peripheral vasodilation, resulting from the vascular α-adrenoceptor blocking action of labetalol. At the same time, in exercising human subjects, blood pressure increments seemed to be blocked to a greater degree than has previously been reported with propranolol, probably because of the concomitant α-adrenergic blockade.[5,19]

At rest, labetalol has been shown not to appreciably lower heart rate and left ventricular stroke volume, in contrast to propranolol, where both these parameters are attenuated, and to phentolamine where they are increased. The effect of labetalol on resting heart rate is most probably reflex in origin, resulting from vagal withdrawal in response to the peripheral vasodilation mediated by α-adrenergic blockade.[5] In exercising human subjects, the increment in heart rate is attenuated by labetalol similarly to propranolol.[5]

The resting cardiac output has been shown not to appreciably decrease with labetalol,[14] an effect which may be mediated by the vasodilating of "unloading" effects of α-adrenergic blockade, in contrast to the decrease in cardiac output seen with propranolol (increased peripheral resistance due to unopposed α-adrenergic-induced vasoconstriction).

With regard to other physiologic parameters, labetalol has been shown to have a lesser bronchoconstrictive effect than propranolol with similar degrees of β-blockade (possibly mediated by α-adrenergic blockade).[5,15] The effects of labetalol in platelet function, hemoglobin-oxygen dissociation, electrophysiologic function, and glucose metabolism have not been well elucidated.

THERAPEUTIC APPLICATIONS AND CLINICAL EXPERIENCE

The hemodynamic profile of action of labetalol suggested its application in cardiovascular disorders such as hypertension, ischemic heart disease, and cardiac arrhythmias.

HYPERTENSION

To date, the major clinical experience with labetalol has been in the treatment of hypertension. β-Adrenoceptor agents, such as propranolol, reduce blood pressure mainly by lowering cardiac output[15] (perhaps also through a central nervous system effect), but do not primarily, or consistently, affect peripheral vascular resistance.[16] β-Adrenoceptor blockers may be effective in some patients with hypertension, but usually must be combined with other antihypertensive agents (e.g., diuretics, vasodilators).[17]

Constriction of the peripheral resistance vessels is mediated through α-adrenoceptors. Pure α-blockers (phentolamine) have not found much clinical application in hypertension because of their unpleasant side effects: reflex tachycardia and orthostatic hypotension.[18] An agent like labetalol which combines the properties of efficient blockade of both the α-adrenoceptors of the resistance vessels and the β-adrenoceptors in the heart can be anticipated to lessen blood pressure by decreasing the peripheral resistance, and, at the same time, inhibit the reflex increase of heart rate and cardiac output.

Labetalol has been shown to be an effective and safe antihypertensive agent in multiple clinical trials to date.[19-30] Short-term intravenous trials with the drug in hypertension (1 to 2 mg per kg) have shown dramatic reductions in both systolic and diastolic blood pressure (usually within 5 to 20 minutes) during rest, while exercise-induced rises in systolic and diastolic pressures were considerably attenuated.[19,27,29,30] Labetalol is the first β-blocker that intravenously has proven effective in hypertensive crises.[31] Although there is a dramatic reduction in blood pressure in the standing position, the incidence of dizziness and syncope has been infrequent (probably because labetalol is not as potent an α-adrenoceptor blocker as phentolamine).

In oral doses of 25 to 3200 mg per day, labetalol has shown to be efficacious both in the short-term and long-term (up to 3 years) management of hypertension.[21,23] Most patients with mild to moderate hypertension responded to doses of 400 to 800 mg per day.[22,26] Postural hypotension and dizziness were usually seen with doses over 2000 mg per day.[23] Drug tolerance does not develop.[23]

In 16 patients resistant to conventional antihypertensive therapy (a multidrug regimen), oral labetalol was effective by itself in normalizing the blood pressure in 10 patients. High doses of drug (range 1200 to 8000 mg per day, mean daily dose 3091 mg), however, were required, with postural hypotension a bothersome side effect necessitating discontinuance of the drug in three subjects.[24]

In controlled comparative trials oral labetalol (800 mg per day) proved more efficacious than oral propranolol (320 mg per day) in management of moderately severe hypertension. Group average heart rates were lower in patients treated with propranolol compared with labetalol. Labetalol caused a greater fall in blood pressure in the standing position and attenuated the exercise induced rise in blood pressure.

In another comparative study, oral labetalol (400 mg per day) proved a more efficacious antihypertensive agent than a combination of oxprenolol-phentolamine.[33] In two comparative intravenous studies in hypertension, labetalol was shown to be more effective than propranolol.[28,34]

Labetalol has been shown to be useful in the medical and surgical management of patients with pheochromocytoma and relieved symptoms in a patient experiencing hypertensive crisis after clonidine withdrawal.[31] The drug was extremely well-tolerated in patients undergoing surgery with halothane anesthesia.[35]

Labetalol is an important new addition to the antihypertensive regimen currently available. As a single drug it has been therapeutically equated with a propranolol-hydralazine combination.[19] It can be used in hypertensive crises without causing the secondary tachycardia seen with diazoxide and hydralazine.[36] Since it does not decrease cardiac stroke volume[21] it may be a useful drug in hypertensive patients with associated coronary and/or cerebral insufficiency.

The major side effects seen in patients treated with labetalol are postural hypotension and dizziness, which are usually self-limited. Some patients cannot tolerate the drug for these reasons, however.[21-26,30,32,33]

The effects of labetalol on renin, angiotensin, and aldosterone levels are not well defined. There is some preliminary evidence that elevated renin levels are attenuated.[19,28]

ISCHEMIC HEART DISEASE

There is very little experience with labetalol in the management of angina pectoris. One study showed the drug to be effective in increasing exercise tolerance in patients with angina.[37] The mechanism of the therapeutic effect of β-blockers in angina pectoris is the reduction of heart rate and blood pressure increments with exercise.[38] Labetalol lowers the heart rate-blood pressure product with exercise and should prove to be clinically efficacious.[19] The unique α-blocking effect of labetalol may also provide new and exciting therapeutic benefits. α-Receptors are present in the coronary arteries and a drug which can block adrenergic tone may increase blood flow while myocardial oxygen demands are being reduced. A study by Maxwell,[39] in dogs, showed that intravenous labetalol increases the coronary blood flow, in contrast to other β-blockers where the opposite effects on coronary blood flow has been demonstrated.[39] Studies are now in progress, in our institution, comparing labetalol to a propranolol-nitrate combination in patients with angina pectoris. With coronary spasm now being recognized as a possible cause for angina pectoris and myocardial infarction, labetalol, with its α-adrenergic properties, might prove to be extremely useful for these indications.[40]

ARRHYTHMIAS

There is very limited clinical experience with labetalol in therapy of cardiac arrhythmias. Since labetalol has β-blocking properties identical to propranolol, it should prove efficacious in those clinical settings where propranolol has proven effective.

CONGESTIVE HEART FAILURE

Labetalol with its α-adrenergic blocking (vasodilating, "unloading properties") might prove efficacious in hypertension, angina pectoris, and arrhythmias with associated mild-to-moderate congestive heart failure, where pure β-adrenoceptor blocking drugs are contraindicated. Preliminary hemodyamic studies in hypertensive patients have shown no deterioration in left ventricular function with therapeutic doses of labetalol.[20,21,27] Clinical studies are now in progress evaluating the efficacy of labetalol as vasodilator therapy in patients with congestive heart failure.

SIDE EFFECTS AND TOXICOLOGY (Table 11-3)

The most common side effect of labetalol is postural dizziness related to postural hypertension.[21-26] In a collected series of 350 patients, this symptom appeared in 3 to 5 percent of patients during initiation of treatment, however, it was self-limited in most instances.[21-34,41] When high doses of the drug are used (2000 mg) this side effect is more commonly seen, with frequent patient intolerance.[22,24] Other side effects, which were rarely noted, were fatigue, nightmares (usually with high doses), nausea, bronchospasm, and nasal stuffiness.

Labetalol binds reversibly to the melanin pigment of the uveal tract of the eye.[13] Unlike the drugs chlorpromazine and chloraquine, no clinical

TABLE 11-3. Adverse Reactions and Toxicity–Collected Series (350 patients)[21-34,41]

Adverse Reactions
1. Postural dizziness (postural hypertension, usually seen with high doses [2000 mg/day])
2. Nasal stuffiness (rare)
3. Fatigue (rare)
4. Nightmares (rare)
5. Bronchospasm (rare)

Toxicity
No clinical toxicity seen to date
1. Occasional antinuclear antibody titre elevation
2. Reversible binding of drug to melanin in uveal tract of eye (no ophthalmologic symptoms)

ophthalmic signs have been demonstrated to date.[13] Continuous clinical observation is necessary, however, because of the oculomucotaneus syndrome that has been seen with another β-blocker, practolol.[42]

Occasional patients have demonstrated positive antinuclear titers, but no associated clinical symptoms have been described.[26]

CONCLUSIONS

Labetalol is the forerunner of a new group of β-adrenoceptor blocking drugs with the properties of combined α- and β-adrenoceptor blockade. The drug has been proven useful in treatment of hypertension with a low incidence of postural hypotension. The potential therapeutic activity of labetalol in angina pectoris and arrhythmia is currently being assessed in worldwide clinical trials.

REFERENCES

1. Ahlquist RP: A study of the adrenotropic receptors. Am J Physiol 153: 586–600, 1948
2. Farmer JB, Kennedy I, Levy GP, Marshall RJ: Pharmacology of AH 5158: a drug which blocks both α and β-adrenoceptors. Br J Pharmacol 45: 660–675, 1972
3. Boakes AJ, Knight EJ, Prichard BNC: Preliminary studies of the pharmacological effects of 5-1-hydroxy-2-(1-methyl-3-phenyl propyl) amino-ethyl salicylamide, AH 5158, in man. Clin Sci 40: 18–20, 1971
4. Collier JG, Dawnay NAH, Nachev CH, Robinson BF: Clinical investigation of an antagonist at α and β-adrenoceptors, AH 5158. Br J Pharmacol 44: 286–293, 1972
5. Brittain RT, Levy GP: A review of the animal pharmacology of labetalol, a combined α and β-adrenoceptor blocking drug. Br J Clin Pharmacol 3 (Suppl 3): 681–694, 1976
6. Richardson PS, Sterling GM: Effects of β-adrenergic receptor blockade on airway conductance and lung volume in normal and asthmatic subjects. Br Med J 3: 143–145, 1969
7. Fleisch JH, Maling HM, Brodie BB: Evidence for existence of alpha-adrenergic receptors in mammalian trachea. Am J Physiol 218: 596–599, 1970
8. Bewtra A, Longo F, Adolphson R, Townley R: Quantitative determination of alpha-adrenergic receptor activity in human trachea in vitro. J Allerg Clin Immunol 55: 93, 1975
9. Patel KR, Kerr JW: Alpha-receptor blocking drugs in bronchial asthma. Lancet 1: 348–349, 1975
10. Geumei A, Miller JR, Miller WF: Effects of phentolamine inhalation on patients with bronchial asthma. Br J Clin Pharmacol 2: 539–540, 1975
11. Coltart DJ, Shand DG: Plasma propranolol levels in the quantitative assessment of β-adrenergic blockade in man. Br Med J 3: 731–734, 1970
12. Martin LE, Hopkins R, Bland R: Metabolism of labetalol by animals and man. Br J Clin Pharmacol 3 (Suppl 3): 695–710, 1976

180

FRISHMAN

13. Poynter D, Martin LE, Harrison C, Cook J: Affinity of labetalol for ocular melanin. Br J Clin Pharmacol 3: (Suppl. 3) 711-720, 1976
14. Koch G: Hemodynamic effects of combined α and β-adrenoceptor blockade after intravenous labetalol in hypertensive patients at rest and during exercise. Br J Clin Pharmacol 3: (Suppl 3) 725-728, 1976
15. Skinner C, Gaddie J, Palmer KNV: Comparison of intravenous AH 5158 (ibidomide) and propranolol in asthma. Br Med J 2: 59-61, 1975
16. Hansson L, Zweifler AJ, Julius S, Hunyor SN: Hemodynamic effects of acute and prolonged β-adrenergic blockade in essential hypertension. Acta Medica Scand 196: 27-34, 1974
17. Zacest R, Gilmore E, Koch-Weber J: Treatment of essential hypertension with combined vasodilation and β-adrenergic blockade. N Engl J Med 286: 617-622, 1972
18. Berlin LJ, Juel-Jensen BE: α and β-adrenoceptor blockade in hypertension. Lancet 1: 979-985, 1972
19. Mehta J, Cohn JN: Hemodynamic effects of labetalol, an alpha and beta adrenergic blocking agent in hypertensive subjects. Circulation 55: 370-375, 1977
20. Koch G: Haemodynamic effects of combined α and β-adrenoceptor blockade after intravenous labetalol in hypertensive patients at rest and during exercise. Br J Clin Pharmacol 3 (Suppl 3): 725-728, 1976
21. Koch G: Combined α and β-adrenoreceptor blockade with oral labetalol in hypertensive patients with reference to haemodynamic effects at rest and during exercise. Br J Clin Pharmacol 3 (Suppl 3): 729-732, 1976
22. Kane J, Gregg I, Richards DA: A double-blind trial of labetalol. Br J Clin Pharmacol 3 (Suppl 3): 737-741, 1976
23. Prichard BNC, Boakes AJ: Labetalol in long-term treatment of hypertension. Br J Clin Pharmacol 3 (Suppl 3): 743-750, 1976
24. Dargie HJ, Dollery CT, Daniel J: Labetalol in resistant hypertension. Br J Clin Pharmacol 3 (Suppl 3): 751-755, 1976
25. Hansson L, Hänel B: Labetalol, and new α- and β-adrenoceptor-blocking agent, in hypertension. Br J Clin Pharmacol 3 (Suppl 3): 763-764, 1976
26. Bolli P, Waal-Manning HJ, Wood AJ, Simpson FO: Experience with labetalol in hypertension. Br J Clin Pharmacol 3 (Suppl 3): 765-771, 1976
27. Joekes AM, Thompson FD: Acute haemodynamic effects of labetalol and its subsequent use as an oral hypotensive agent. Br J Clin Pharmacol 3 (Suppl 3): 789-793, 1976
28. Trust PM, Rosei EA, Brown JJ, et al.: Effect of blood pressure, angiotensin II and aldosterone concentrations during treatment of severe hypertension with intravenous labetalol: comparison with propranolol. Br J Clin Pharmacol 3 (Suppl 3): 799-803, 1976
29. Ronne-Rasmussen JO, Andersen GS, Bowal Jensen N, Andersson E: Acute effect of intravenous labetalol in the treatment of systemic arterial hypertension. Br J Clin Pharmacol 3 (Suppl 3): 805-808, 1976
30. Pearson RM, Havard CWH: Intravenous labetalol in hypertensive patients treated with β-adrenoceptor-blocking drugs. Br J Clin Pharmacol 3 (Suppl 3): 795-798, 1976
31. Rosei EA, Brown JJ, Lever AF, et al.: Treatment of phaeochromocytoma and of clonidine withdrawal hypertension with labetalol. Br J Clin Pharmacol 3 (Suppl 3): 809-815, 1976

32. Pugsley DJ, Armstrong BK, Nassim MA, Beilin LJ: Controlled comparison of labetalol and propranolol in the management of severe hypertension. Br J Clin Pharmacol 3 (Suppl 3): 777–782, 1976

33. Johnson BF, LaBrooy J, Munro-Faure AD: Comparative anti-hypertensive effects of labetalol and the combination of oxprenolol and phentolamine. Br J Clin Pharmacol 3 (Suppl 3): 783–787, 1976

34. Rosei EA, Trust PM, Brown JJ, et al.: Effects of intravenous labetalol on blood pressure, angiotensin II and aldosterone in hypertension: comparison with propranolol. Clin Sci Mol Med 51: 497–499, 1976

35. Scott DB, Buckley FP, Drummond GB, Littlewood DG, Macrae WR: Cardiovascular effects of labetalol during halothane anesthesia. Br J Clin Pharmacol 3 (Suppl 3): 817–821, 1976

36. Tarazi RC, Dustan HP, Bravo EL, Niarchos AP: Vasodilating drugs: contrasting haemodynamic effects. Clin Sci Mol Med 51: 575–578, 1976

37. Boakes AJ, Prichard BNC: The effect of AH 5158, pindolol, propranolol, and D-propranolol on acute exercise tolerance in angina pectoris. Br J Pharmacol 47: 673–674, 1973

38. Shinebourne E, Fleming J, Hamer J, Prichard BNC: Hemodynamic studies in hypertensive patients treated by oral propranolol. Br Heart J 32: 236–240, 1970

39. Maxwell GM: Effects of alpha- and beta-adrenoceptor antagonist (AH 5158) upon general and coronary hemodynamics of intact dogs. Br J Pharmacol 44: 370–372, 1973

40. Maseri A, L'Abbate A, Baroldi G, et al.: Coronary vasospasm as a possible cause of myocardial infarction. N Engl J Med 299: 1271–1278, 1978

41. Jennings K, Parsons V: A study of labetalol in patients of European, West Indian and West African origin. Br J Clin Pharmacol 3 (Suppl 3): 773–775, 1976

42. Wright P: Untoward effect associated with practolol administration. Oculomucotaneous syndrome. Br Med J 1: 595–598, 1975

CHAPTER TWELVE

Effects of Oral Labetalol in Patients with Both Angina Pectoris and Hypertension

A PRELIMINARY EXPERIENCE

William H. Frishman, Stanley Halprin, Marc Kirschner,
Joel Strom, Marcia Poland, and Edmund Sonnenblick

BETA-ADRENOCEPTOR blocking drugs are widely accepted for the treatment of hypertension, arrhythmias, and angina pectoris.[1,2] Labetalol, 5- (1-hydroxy-2-[(1-methyl-3-phenylpropyl) amino] ethyl) salicylamide (Fig. 12-1) is recently developed and, like propranolol, blocks both β_1 and β_2 vascular and bronchial receptors.[3,4] However, labetalol is unique in that it also has α-adrenergic blocking properties and direct vasodilating activity.[3-5] The β-blocking potency of labetalol is 4 to 16 times that of its α-blocking potency.[3]

α-Adrenergic blocking drugs have limited therapeutic application compared to β-blockers. This may be, in part, because of the unwanted effects of reflex tachycardia and orthostatic hypotension which can aggravate coronary artery disease. In selected patients with variant angina, α-blocking agents have been useful as adjunctive therapy.[6] Patients with coronary artery disease develop increased cardiovascular resistance following the cold pres-

LABETALOL

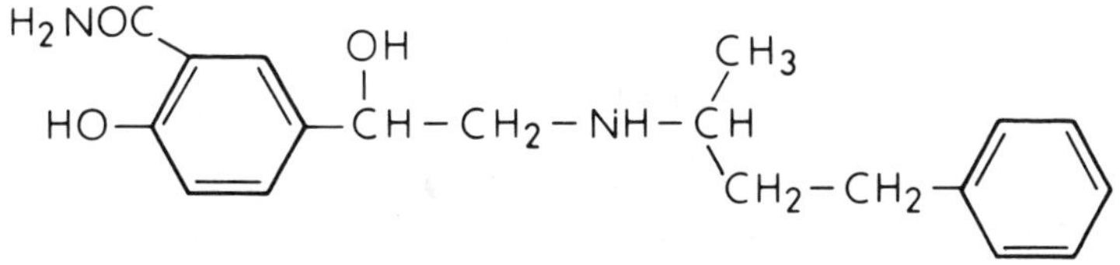

Figure 12-1.   Chemical structure of labetalol.

sor test.[7] Phentolamine reverses these effects. This latter finding raises the possibility that α-adrenoceptor blockade may play a role in the prevention of myocardial ischemia.[7,8]

Labetalol, a β- α-blocker, has been shown to be a potent antihypertensive drug.[4,9–13] Intravenous administration of labetalol in patients with angina pectoris resulted in a marked increase in exercise tolerance.[14] In the present pilot study, the effects of oral labetalol in patients who have both angina pectoris and essential hypertension were assessed.

METHODS

PATIENTS

Six male patients with stable angina pectoris and systemic hypertension were entered in the study. The average age was 55 years (range 47–59 years). The diagnosis of angina pectoris was established by clinical history (symptoms and response to sublingual nitroglycerin) and the development of typical angina pectoris with the treadmill exercise test. In addition, 5 of the 6 patients had an exercise induced ECG ST-segment depression of at least 1 mm of the ischemic type. The diagnosis of coronary artery disease was made by coronary angiography in three patients (a stenosis compromising the lumen of at least one major coronary artery by more than 75 percent) and by a previously documented myocardial infarction in the other three. All patients had to have at least five attacks of angina pectoris a week for one month with no evidence for an accelerated course. Hypertension was documented in all patients by an average 3-minute standing diastolic pressure of $\geq 90 \leq 110$ mm Hg (using Korotkoff Phase V) on at least two separate outpatient visits while untreated.

Patients with the following conditions were excluded from the study: coexistent valvular heart disease, congestive heart failure, bronchial asthma, severe bradycardia, (resting heart rate <50 beats per minute), intermittent claudication, and either myocardial infarction or coronary artery bypass within three months.

None of the patients received medication during the trial other than the study drug and sublingual nitroglycerin. Written informed consent was obtained in all instances.

EXPERIMENTAL DESIGN

This study was divided into three periods. A 3-week placebo period in which patients received placebo* three times daily (tid) was followed by a

* Schering Corporation, Bloomfield, New Jersey 07003

4-week labetalol treatment period. The dose of labetalol was titrated weekly (100 to 400 mg tid) to achieve the optimal antihypertensive effect and improvement in the patient's anginal symptoms. The optimal antihypertensive effect was defined as an average 3-minute standing diastolic blood pressure of <90 mm Hg and at least a 10 mm Hg reduction from placebo baseline. Improvement in angina was defined by a significant decrease in the number of anginal attacks and a significant increase in exercise tolerance. If the antihypertensive goal is achieved at a lower dose than the maximum, but the angina did not improve, the dose of labetalol was to be increased. This increase was only to be made if it was felt that the patient could tolerate it without developing clinical signs of hypotension, however. At the end of this 4-week therapeutic period, the dose of labetalol was tapered over a 2-day interval. The patient was reassessed 1 to 4 days after cessation of labetalol and again in one week.

METHODS OF OBSERVATION

All patients kept a detailed daily record of the angina attacks they experienced, the number of nitroglycerin tablets taken, and an estimation of the physical activity for that day. Every week, the patients were evaluated with a detailed history and physical examination which included measurements of supine and standing (3 minute) heart rate and blood pressure. Blood pressure and heart rate determinations were always made 2 hours after ingestion of placebo or labetalol, which is the time of the peak pharmacologic effect of labetalol.[15] Patients also underwent multistage treadmill exercise studies (Bruce-Protocol)[16] each week. Complete blood counts, urinalyses, chest roentgenograms, resting electrocardiograms, and biochemical blood screening tests (total protein, albumin, calcium, phosphate, cholesterol, triglycerides, uric acid, blood urea nitrogen, glucose, sodium, potassium, chloride, total bilirubin, alkaline phosphatase, SGOT, SGPT, CPK, LDH, CO_2) were performed pre- and postlabetalol treatment.

EXERCISE TESTS

Multistage exercise testing following the Bruce protocol[16] was performed weekly with the use of a treadmill. The blood pressure was measured every minute during exercise by the auscultory method and the ECG monitored on the oscilloscope. The endpoint of exercise was angina pectoris defined by the patient's typical chest pain discomfort. An abnormal electrocardiographic response was defined as a flat or downsloping ST-segment depression of 1 mm of 0.08 seconds duration after the terminus of the QRS complex with the P-Ta segment as the baseline of reference.

Work performance was expressed in total minutes of treadmill exercise. The product of heart rate and systolic blood pressure, an indirect index of myocardial oxygen consumption,[17] was calculated from measurements obtained at each 1-minute measuring interval.

STATISTICAL ANALYSIS

Group means are presented with the standard error of the mean as the index of dispersion. Comparisons between treatment phases were made using Student's paired two-tailed t test.

RESULTS

EFFECTS ON RESTING BLOOD PRESSURE AND HEART RATE (Table 12-1)

There was a statistically significant reduction in supine and standing systolic and diastolic blood pressures from placebo baseline (Fig. 12-2). After 4 weeks of labetalol treatment, mean supine systolic blood pressure was reduced by 23.4 mm Hg and the standing systolic blood pressure fell by 33 mm Hg. While there was a postural fall in systolic pressure, this was not statistically significant. Mean supine diastolic blood pressure was reduced

TABLE 12-1.   Effects of Labetalol on Resting Heart Rate and Blood Pressure in Patients with Both Angina Pectoris and Hypertension

	Baseline (Placebo) N = 6	Peak Dose Labetalol (Mean Dose: 950 mg) N = 6	Difference	Significance
Supine				
Heart rate (beats/min)	76.8 ±4.7*	63.9 ±3.5	−12.9 ±2.5	p < 0.005
Systolic BP (mm Hg)	158.8 ±4.0	135.3 ±9.9	−23.5 ±4.5	p < 0.005
Diastolic BP (mm Hg)	103.64 ±1.6	87.1 ±2.1	−16.5 ±3.6	p < 0.01
3-Minute Standing				
Heart rate (beats/min)	75.9 ±5.1	67.7 ±3.1	−8.2 ±4.3	Not significant
Systolic BP (mm Hg)	154.6 ±6.1	121.6 ±7.9	−33.0 ±5.7	p < 0.005
Diastolic BP (mm Hg)	102.0 ±1.7	83.1 ±4.1	−18.9 ±3.1	p < 0.005

*Mean ± standard error of the mean.

by 16.5 mm Hg and standing diastolic blood pressure by 18.9 mm Hg. Supine heart rate fell by 12.9 beats per minute which was statistically significant ($p < 0.005$). The standing heart rate was approximately 5 beats per minute higher than the supine heart rate. The standing heart rate fell 8.3 beats per minute, but this was not a statistically significant fall.

EFFECTS ON ANGINA PECTORIS

Subjective improvement was found in a significant reduction ($p < 0.05$)

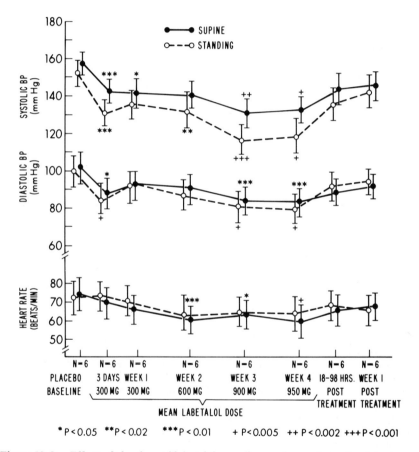

Figure 12-2. Effects of placebo and labetalol on resting, supine, and standing blood pressure and heart rate. Compared to placebo, a significant decrease in systolic and diastolic blood pressure is seen with initiation of labetalol therapy (300 mg per day), an effect which is augmented when higher doses of the drug are used. A significant decrease in supine heart rate is seen with labetalol, 600 to 900 mg per day, compared to placebo. There is no rebound in heart rate and blood pressure above placebo values one week postwithdrawal.

in the number of angina pectoris attacks (and nitroglycerin consumption) per week (8.5 ±2.6 attacks at baseline and 1.0 ±0.6 attacks after 4 weeks of labetalol treatment). The quality of life of the patients was enhanced; they reported increased ability to perform activities of daily living. All patients were Functional Class III (American Heart Association Criteria) on entry into the study and became Class II after 4 weeks of labetalol.

STRESS TEST RESULTS (Table 12-2 and Fig. 12-3)

The resting heart rate prior to the exercise stress test was decreased from placebo baseline by 10 ±3.5 beats per minute, which was statistically significant ($p < 0.02$). The heart rate was also significantly reduced at Stage I ($p < 0.02$) of the Bruce Protocol, but not at Stage II. While there was an absolute reduction in heart rate, there was no inhibition of the exercise-induced increases in heart rate, as measured by the beats per minute increase in heart rate from rest to Stage I and II, at baseline and after 4 weeks of labetalol. The peak heart rate achieved with exercise after labetalol therapy was not significantly different from placebo baseline, even though total exercise time increased by 45 percent.

TABLE 12-2.   Effects of Labetalol on Exercise Tolerance and Determinants of Myocardial Oxygen Consumption

	Baseline (placebo)	Peak Dose Labetalol (mean dose: 950 mg)	Difference	Significance
Exercise time (min, N = 6)	4.3 ±0.9*	6.3 ±0.4	+2.0 ±0.6	p < 0.02
Exercise peak systolic pressure (mm Hg, N = 6)	188.3 ±18.9	148.3 ±17.8	−38.3 ±7.0	p < 0.005
Exercise peak heart rate (beats/min, N = 6)	124.5 ±9.9	118.0 ±6.2	−6.5 ±5.1	NS
Exercise peak heart RPP (N = 6)	23,708 ±3376	17,705 ±2560	−6003 ±1600	p < 0.02
Heart rate change from rest to Stage I (beats/min, N = 6)	34.7 ±6.6	29.5 ±3.5	−5.2 ±5.3	NS
Heart rate change from rest to Stage II (beats/min, N = 4)	42.0 ±7.9	41.3 ±4.7	−0.7 ±3.9	NS
Systolic blood pressure change from rest to Stage I (N = 6)	15.5 ±7.9	5.0 ±3.9	−10.5 ±6.3	NS
Systolic blood pressure change from rest to Stage II (N = 4)	38.7 ±11.3	16.8 ±9.9	−22.0 ±5.6	p < 0.05

**Mean ± standard error of the mean.*

   The resting systolic blood pressure prior to the stress test was significantly reduced (p < 0.001), as was the systolic blood pressure at Stage I and
II (p < 0.005). However, a significant inhibition of exercise-induced increases in systolic blood pressure was found only at Stage II (p < 0.05); no
significant inhibition was found at Stage I. At Stage I, the mean reduction
in the rise from rest with placebo to the rise after labetalol was −10.5 mm Hg
and the significant inhibition at Stage II was −22.0 mm Hg.

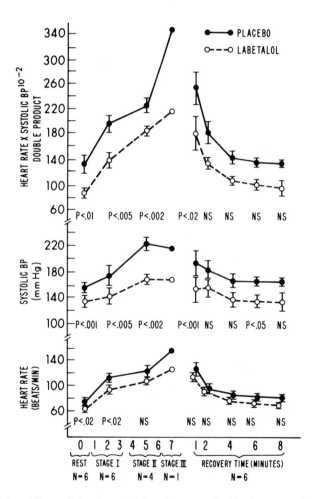

Figure 12-3. Effects of placebo and labetalol on systolic blood pressure, heart rate, and
rate-pressure product during rest, exercise, and recovery. Systolic blood pressure, heart rate,
and rate-pressure product with exercise (Stage I — Bruce) are significantly lower in labetalol treated patients when compared to placebo. Following exercise, the time for recovery to
baseline heart rate and blood pressure is similar with placebo and labetalol.

With significant reductions in both heart rate and systolic blood pressure, it is not surprising that the rate pressure product (heart rate × systolic blood pressure) is also significantly reduced at rest and during exercise following labetalol treatment ($p < 0.02$). It should be noted that even though the peak rate pressure product is significantly less ($p < 0.02$) than at placebo baseline, the patients had a significant increase in their exercise tolerance.

At the end point of the stress test, there was no significant decrease in the magnitude of the ST-segment depression. It should be remembered that exercise time significantly increased, however. These findings are best illustrated in a patient with 3 vessel coronary artery involvement (Fig 12-4).

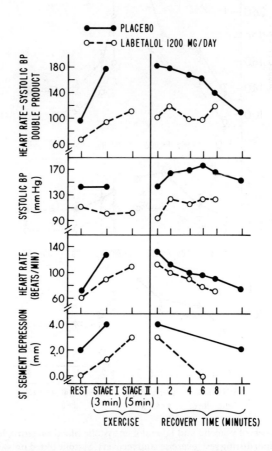

Figure 12-4. The effects of placebo and labetalol on systolic blood pressure, heart rate, rate-pressure product, and ECG ST-segment depression, during rest, exercise, and recovery in a representative patient (C.M.).

EFFECTS OF LABETALOL WITHDRAWAL
(Table 12-3, Fig. 12-3)

One week following labetalol withdrawal, there was a return of resting blood pressure, heart rate, and rate pressure product towards placebo values without evidence of rebound. Though not significant, because of a high variability, the mean values following withdrawal were lower than at placebo baseline.

TABLE 12-3.   Effects of Labetalol Withdrawal (1 Week Posttherapy) on Blood Pressure and Heart Rate Compared to Control

	Baseline (Placebo) N = 6	Labetalol Withdrawal (1 Week Posttherapy)	Difference†
Supine			
Heart rate (beats/min)	76.8 ±4.7*	71.4 ±3.4	−5.4 ±6.0
Systolic BP (mm Hg)	158.8 ±4.0	149.0 ±4.6	−9.8 ±5.9
Diastolic BP (mm Hg)	103.6 ±1.6	95.8 ±4.4	−7.8 ±4.7
3-Minute standing			
Heart rate (beats/min)	75.9 ±5.1	72.5 ±4.6	−3.4 ±6.1
Systolic BP (mm Hg)	154.6 ±6.1	144.9 ±8.9	−9.7 ±6.8
Diastolic BP (mm Hg)	102.0 ±1.7	97.2 ±5.4	−4.8 ±4.6

*Mean ± standard error of the mean.
†All differences were not significant.

An increase in the frequency of anginal attacks and a reduction in exercise tolerance occurred following withdrawal when compared to the labetalol treatment phase. No patients developed unstable angina pectoris, or an acute myocardial infarction during the one-week withdrawal interval.

ADVERSE EXPERIENCES

Two patients complained of mild dizziness within one day of initiating labetalol treatment, a reaction that was self-limited and not seen later with higher doses. One patient complained of mild fatigue at the highest labetalol dose, which disappeared when the dose was reduced; this same patient complained of decreased libido without ejaculatory dysfunction.

Fundoscopic examinations did not detect any sign of oculotoxicity during the trial.

No abnormalities were found in the hematologic profile, or in liver and renal function tests. There was no significant differences between triglyceride and cholesterol levels after labetalol treatment when compared with placebo.

DISCUSSION

Labetalol, a unique β-adrenergic blocking agent with α-adrenergic blocking properties, is the forerunner of a new pharmacologic class of compounds. β-Adrenergic drugs have an established position in the treatment of essential hypertension and angina pectoris.[1,2] Recent evidence suggests that α-adrenergic blockade may play a role in the prevention of myocardial ischemia by inhibiting neurogenic vasoconstriction in coronary arteries.[8,18-20] Reflex tachycardia and orthostatic hypotension have precluded their use as the sole agent in angina pectoris.[21] Thus, there is a potential advantage to the use of labetalol in the treatment of angina pectoris.

Labetalol is an antihypertensive agent of considerable potency,[9-13] and appears to be more effective than propranolol in reducing blood pressure.[22,23] Labetalol has been shown to be efficacious in hypertensive crises,[24] pheochromocytoma,[25] and in many cases of drug resistant hypertension.[26]

Despite its widespread application in hypertensive disease, there has been little experience in patients with angina pectoris. When administered intravenously to patients with angina pectoris, it produced a significant increase in exercise tolerance, but without any clear cut dose-response relationship.[14] Normotensive patients with coronary artery disease, receiving 200 mg of labetalol daily, demonstrated increased exercise tolerance and electrocardiographic evidence of improvement when compared with placebo.[27]

The results of our preliminary study show that oral labetalol is an effective therapy for patients with both angina pectoris and hypertension. The drug reduced resting systolic and diastolic blood pressure, both supine and standing, upon initiation of therapy (100 mg tid). An augmentation of the antihypertensive effect was seen with higher doses (200 to 400 mg tid). Unlike pure α-adrenergic blocking agents,[21] labetalol reduced the blood pressure without increasing the heart rate. There was a slight reduction in standing heart rate and a significant reduction in supine heart rate. The effects of the drug on systolic blood pressure were more pronounced in the standing position. The differences between standing and supine systolic blood pressure determinations following labetalol may relate to the vasodilatory effects of α-adrenergic blockade which are more important in the standing position. Supine heart rate is significantly reduced while standing heart rate is not. The differences between standing and supine heart rate determinations following labetalol may relate to a compensatory increase in rate with erect posture. Postural hypotension was not seen with labetalol, probably because the drug is a relatively weak α-adrenergic blocker compared to phentolamine. It follows, then, that the components of the reduction in rate-pressure product with labetalol in the supine and standing positions differ: In the upright position, there is a greater reduction in systolic blood pressure and a lesser reduction in heart rate. In the supine position, on the other hand, there is a lesser reduction in systolic blood pressure and a greater reduction in heart rate.

There was a significant reduction in spontaneous attacks of angina pectoris and a significant increase in exercise tolerance with the peak labetalol dose.

At a comparable level of exercise (Stage I — Bruce), the heart rate, blood pressure, and rate-pressure product (an indirect measure of myocardial oxygen consumption)[17] in patients treated with labetalol were reduced. The peak heart rate-blood pressure product achieved with exercise was lower following labetalol than it was with placebo, despite a marked increase in exercise tolerance. Thus, in this small series, labetalol appears to be an effective antianginal agent, increasing exercise tolerance while reducing myocardial oxygen demands.

There were no intolerable adverse reactions noted with the drug, and one week following labetalol withdrawal there was no hyperadrenergic rebound state demonstrable. Following withdrawal, the heart rate and blood pressure were slightly lower (not significantly) than baseline placebo levels (although significantly higher than with labetalol). This might reflect a prolonged action of the drug despite its short plasma half-life,[15] or a training effect in the patients.

Beyond the improvement in exercise tolerance and reduction in angina attacks, there are other potential therapeutic advantages in the use of α-β-adrenoceptor blocking agents in angina pectoris. Since neurogenic vasoconstrictor impulses to the coronary-resistance vessels are transmitted through sympathetic nerves acting upon α-adrenergic receptors in the coronary vascular bed, there may be an important role for α-adrenergic blocking drugs in the prevention of coronary spasm and in the preservation of restricted coronary blood flow.[6-8,18-20,28-31] This was suggested in a study by Mudge et al.,[7] in which phentolamine was shown to block reflex coronary vasoconstriction regularly elicited by the cold-pressor test. Orlick et al.[6] also demonstrated that α-adrenergic blockade was a useful adjunct in selected patients with variant angina.

β-Adrenoceptor blocking drugs have been shown to decrease coronary blood flow in patients.[8,30] Stimulation of β_2-receptors, which induced vasodilation in coronary arteries, can be blocked by propranolol.[32] Indeed, blockade with nonselective β-adrenergic blockers may actually be detrimental in patients in whom ischemia is due to reduced oxygen delivery secondary to coronary spasm.[32] Nonselective β-adrenoceptor blockade may allow the unopposed influence of coronary vasoconstrictor impulses to prevail. Coronary blood flow was found to increase following intravenous labetalol administration in dogs.[33] Labetalol, with its α-adrenergic properties, may increase coronary blood flow, while at the same time reducing myocardial oxygen demands in man.

Labetalol may also have applicability in situations where other β-adrenergic blocking drugs are contraindicated. α-Adrenergic hypersensitivity has been shown to be important in many cases of bronchial asthma, suggesting that the α-adrenergic blocking activity of labetalol may be beneficial.[34-39] In asthmatic patients with angina pectoris, Skinner and his associates[40] found that propranolol, administered intravenously, produced bronchoconstriction in asthmatics. Labetalol, in equivalent cardiac β-adrenoceptor blocking doses, did not cause bronchoconstriction. Labetalol also lowers peripheral vascular resistance while other β-adrenergic blockers elevate resistance.[41] With its afterload reducing effects, labetalol may be an ideal drug for patients with angina pectoris and hypertension associated with occult or mild congestive heart failure.

CONCLUSIONS

In this pilot study, labetalol was a safe and effective agent for reducing spontaneous attacks of angina pectoris, improving exercise tolerance, and reducing high blood pressure. There are still many unanswered questions, however. Double-blind studies need to be initiated in patients with angina pectoris comparing labetalol to other β-adrenergic blocking agents, nitrates, and placebo. The effects of labetalol on left ventricular function, platelets, and coronary blood flow in humans need to be elucidated. The effects of labetalol in normotensive patients with angina pectoris also must be examined.

Labetalol is an important pharmacologic advance that provides an entirely new concept in management of patients with angina pectoris and hypertension: α-β-adrenergic blockade.

SUMMARY

The safety and efficacy of oral labetalol, an α-β-adrenergic blocking drug, was assessed in six patients with both angina pectoris and essential hypertension. Patients received a placebo for three weeks which was followed by a 4-week titration of labetalol (100 to 400 mg tid). The dose was then withdrawn over a 2-day period. With maximum doses of labetalol, exercise tolerance as measured by multistage treadmill testing, increased significantly compared to placebo, (p < 0.02). At each exercise level (stage), the heart rate, systolic blood pressure, and rate-pressure product were reduced with labetalol treatment. There was no inhibition of exercise induced increases in heart rate, however, significant inhibition of the systolic pressure increment was seen at stage II (p < 0.05). While peak heart rate was not significantly different from baseline, the peak systolic blood pressure and rate-pressure product were significantly reduced (p < 0.02). Labetalol treatment significantly reduced the number of weekly spontaneous angina attacks (p < 0.05). The resting supine and standing systolic and diastolic blood pressure were significantly reduced by labetalol (p < 0.01). There was no significant reduction in the standing heart rate, but supine heart rate was significantly reduced (p < 0.005). There was no rebound hyperadrenergic effects following labetalol withdrawal. When used alone in patients with both angina pectoris and systemic hypertension, oral labetalol is a safe and effective drug for reducing the symptoms of angina pectoris, improving exercise tolerance, and lowering high blood pressure.

REFERENCES

1. Frishman W, Silverman R: Clinical pharmacology of the new beta adrenergic blocking drugs. Part 2. Physiologic and metabolic effects. Am Heart J 97: 797, 1979
2. Frishman W, Silverman R: Clinical pharmacology of the new beta adrenergic blocking drugs. Part 3. Comparative clinical experience and new therapeutic applications. Am Heart J 98: 119, 1979
3. Brittain RT, Levy GP: A review of the animal pharmacology of labetalol, a combined α and β-adrenoceptor blocking drug. Br J Clin Pharmacol 3 (Suppl 3): 681–694, 1976
4. Frishman W, Halprin S: Clinical pharmacology of the new beta adrenergic blocking drugs. Part 7. New horizons in beta-adrenoceptor blockade therapy: Labetalol. Am Heart J 98: 660–665, 1979
5. Johnson GL, Prioli NA, Ehrreich SJ: Anti-hypertensive effects of labetalol. Fed Proc 36: 1049, 1977 (Abs)
6. Orlick AE, Ricci DR, Cipriano P, Guthaner D, Harrison DC: The role of alpha adrenergic receptors in the pathogenesis of coronary artery spasm. Clin Res 25: 456, 1977
7. Mudge GH Jr, Grossman W, Mills RMJ, Lesch M, Braunwald E: Reflex increase in coronary vascular resistance in patients with ischemic heart disease. N Engl J Med 295: 1333, 1976
8. Hillis LD, Braunwald E: Coronary artery spasm. N Engl J Med 299: 695, 1978
9. Mehta J, Cohn JN: Hemodynamic effects of labetalol, an alpha and beta adrenergic blocking agent in hypertensive subjects. Circulation 55: 370–375, 1977
10. Koch G: Haemodynamic effects of combined α and β-adrenoceptor blockade after intravenous labetalol in hypertensive patients at rest and during exercise. Br J Clin Pharmacol 3 (Suppl 3): 725–728, 1976
11. Prichard BNC, Boakes AJ: Labetalol in long-term treatment of hypertension. Br J Clin Pharmacol 3 (Suppl 3): 743–750, 1976
12. Bolli P, Waal-Manning HJ, Wood AJ, Simpson FO: Experience with labetalol in hypertension. Br J Clin Pharmacol 3 (Suppl 3): 765–771, 1976
13. Joekes AM, Thompson FD: Acute haemodynamic effects of labetalol and its subsequent use as an oral hypotensive agent. Br J Clin Pharmacol 3 (Suppl 3): 789–793, 1976
14. Boakes AJ, Prichard BNC: The effect of AH 5158, pindolol, propranolol, d-propranolol on acute exercise tolerance in angina pectoris. Br J Pharmacol 47: 673, 1973

15. Martin LE, Hopkins R, Bland R: Metabolism of labetalol by animals and man. Br J Clin Pharmacol 3 (Suppl 3): 695–710, 1976
16. Bruce RA: Progress in exercise cardiology. In Yu PN, Goodwin JF (eds): Progress in Cardiology, Vol 3. Philadelphia, Lea and Febiger, 1974, p 113
17. Robinson BF: The mode of action of beta-antagonists in angina pectoris. Circulation 35: 1073, 1967
18. Schwartz PJ, Stone HL: Tonic influence of the sympathetic nervous system on myocardial reactive hyperemia and on coronary blood flow distribution in dogs. Circ Res 41: 51, 1977
19. Mohrman DE, Feigl EO: Competition between sympathetic vasoconstriction and metabolic vasodilation in the canine coronary circulation. Circ Res 42: 79, 1978
20. Murray PA, Vatner SF: Alpha receptor attenuation of coronary vascular response to severe, spontaneous exercise. Fed Proc 37: 235, 1978
21. Berlin LJ, Juel-Jensen BE: α- and β-adrenoceptor blockade in hypertension. Lancet 1: 979–985, 1972
22. Pugsley DJ, Armstrong BK, Nassim MA, Beilin LJ: Controlled comparison of labetalol and propranolol in the management of severe hypertension. Br J Clin Pharmacol 3 (Suppl 3): 777–782, 1976
23. Trust PM, Rosei EA, Brown JJ, et al.: Effect of blood pressure, angiotensin II and aldosterone concentrations during treatment of severe hypertension with intravenous labetalol: comparison with propranolol. Br J Clin Pharmacol 3 (Suppl 3): 799, 1976
24. Ronne-Rasmussen JO, Andersen GS, Bowal Jensen N, Andersson E: Acute effect of intravenous labetalol in the treatment of systemic arterial hypertension. Br J Clin Pharmacol 3 (Suppl 3): 805, 1976
25. Rosei EA, Brown JJ, Lever AF, et al.: Treatment of phaeochromocytoma and of clonidine withdrawal hypertension with labetalol. Br J Clin Pharmacol 3 (Suppl 3): 809, 1976
26. Dargie HJ, Dollery CT, Daniel J: Labetalol in resistant hypertension. Br J Clin Pharmacol 3 (Suppl 3): 751, 1976
27. Brevetti G, Chiariello M, Renyo F, et al.: Labetalol in coronary artery disease. VIII World Congress of Cardiology 1: 194, 1978
28. Pitt B, Elliot EC, Gregg DE: Adrenergic receptor activity in the coronary arteries of the unanesthetized dog. Circ Res 21: 75–84, 1967
29. Levene DL, Freeman MR: Alpha-adrenoceptor mediated coronary artery spasm. JAMA 236: 1018, 1976
30. Rubio R, Berne R: Regulation of coronary blood flow. Prog Cardiovasc Dis 28: 105, 1975
31. Klocke FJ, Mates RE, Copley DP, Orlick AE: Physiology of the coronary circulation in health and coronary artery disease. In Yu P, Goodwin JF (eds): Progress in Cardiology, Vol. 5. Philadelphia, Lea and Febiger, 1976 p 1
32. Braunwald E: Coronary artery spasm and acute myocardial infarction — new possibility for treatment and prevention. N Engl J Med 299: 1101, 1978
33. Maxwell GM: Effects of alpha- and beta-adrenoceptor antagonist (AH 5158) upon general and coronary hemodynamics of intact dogs. Br J Pharmacol 44: 370–372, 1973
34. Richardson PS, Sterling GM: Effects of β-adrenergic receptor blockade on airway conductance and lung volume in normal and asthmatic subjects. Br Med J 3: 143–145, 1969
35. Fleisch JH, Maling HM, Brodie BB: Evidence for existence of alpha-adrenergic receptors in mammalian trachea. Am J Physiol 218: 596, 1970

36. Bewtra A, Longo F, Adolphson R, Townley R: Quantitative determination of alpha-adrenergic receptor activity in human trachea *in vitro*. J Allerg Clin Immunol 55: 93, 1975
37. Patel KR, Kerr JW: Alpha-receptor blocking drugs in bronchial asthma. Lancet 1: 348–349, 1975
38. Geumei A, Miller JR, Miller WF: Effects of phentolamine inhalation on patients with bronchial asthma. Br J Clin Pharmacol 2: 539–540, 1975
39. Henderson WR, Shelhamer JH, Reingold DB, et al.: Alpha-adrenergic hyperresponsiveness in asthma. N Engl J Med 300: 642, 1979
40. Skinner C, Gaddie J, Palmer KNV: Comparison of intravenous AH 5158 (ibidomide) and propranolol in asthma. Br Med J 2: 59–61, 1975
41. Sweet CS, Solar J, Gaul SL: Peripheral vasodilator and β-adrenoceptor blocking properties of several β-adrenoceptor antagonists. Clin Exper Hyper 1: 449, 1979

CHAPTER THIRTEEN

The Beta-Adrenergic Blocking Drugs: A Perspective

William H. Frishman

THE introduction of β-adrenoceptor blocking drugs to the armamendarium of clinical medicine has provided one of the major therapeutic advances of this century. The pioneers in this field hypothesized that β-adrenergic blockade would be beneficial in patients with angina pectoris; this assumption has now been proven beyond doubt. These pioneers could not have foreseen the large spectrum of therapeutic indications that are now being discovered[1-60] (Table 13-1). β-Adrenoceptor blocking agents have been found to be efficacious in neuropsychiatric disorders, endocrine disor-

TABLE 13-1. **Reported Cardiovascular Indications for** β**-Adrenoceptor Blocking Drugs**

1. Hypertension[1, 2]
2. Angina pectoris[3, 4]
3. Arrhythmias[5, 6]
4. Myocardial infarction[7, 8]
5. Dissection of the aorta[9, 10]
6. Hypertrophic cardiomyopathy[11, 12]
7. Digitalis intoxication[13]
8. Mitral valve prolapse[14]
9. "QT Interval" prolongation syndrome[15]
10. Tetralogy of Fallot[16]
11. Mitral stenosis[17, 18]
12. Cardiogenic shock[19]
13. Fetal tachycardia[20]
14. Neurocirculatory asthenia[21]
15. Pulmonary stenosis and atresia[22, 23]
16. Erythromelalgia[24]
17. Hypertensive response with endotracheal intubation[25]
18. Hypertensive response with human coitus[26]

ders, as well as disorders of other organ systems (Table 13-2). There is little doubt that the list of therapeutic indications in all the subspecialty areas of medicine will continue to lengthen as a result of the fecund inventiveness of clinical investigators. At this juncture, β-adrenoceptor blocking drugs have been approved by the U.S. FDA for the treatment of angina pectoris (propranolol, timolol, nadolol), hypertension (propranolol, timolol, nadolol, pindolol, metoprolol), arrhythmias (propranolol), migraine prophylaxis (propranolol), and glaucoma (timolol).

TABLE 13-2. Reported Noncardiovascular Indications for β-Adrenoceptor Blocking Drugs

Neuropsychiatric
1. Migraine[27]
2. Parkinson's disease[28]
3. Essential tremor[29]
4. Anxiety[30]
5. "Exam nerves"[31]
6. Alcohol withdrawal (delerium tremens)[32]
7. Narcotic withdrawal[33]
8. Cocaine toxicity[34]
9. LSD-induced anxiety states[35]
10. Schizophrenia[36]
11. Lithium-induced tremor[37]
12. Narcolepsy[38]

Endocrine
13. Thyrotoxicosis[39, 40]
14. Hyperparathyroidism[41, 42]
15. Insulinoma[43]
16. Unstable juvenile diabetes mellitus[44]
17. Renal osteodystrophy[45]

Other
18. Glaucoma[46]
19. Tetanus[47]
20. Acne vulgaris[48]
21. Acute prophyria[49]
22. Endotoxin shock[50]
23. Hemorrhagic shock[51]
24. Ureteral colic[52]
25. Urinary incontinence[53]
26. Phantom limb[54]
27. Bile acid-induced diarrhea[55]
28. Spastic colon[56]
29. Dysfunctional labor[57]
30. Hypothermia and hypoxia[58]
31. Disseminated intravascular coagulation[59]
32. Oleander poisoning[60]

Within the next 5 years, other β-adrenoceptor blocking agents, with cardioselectivity, partial agonist effects, α-adrenergic blocking activity, and prolonged pharmacologic half-lives, may be approved. For the major cardiac indications (hypertension, arrhythmias, angina pectoris), no one β-blocker has been shown to be more efficacious than another.[61, 62] However, the differing pharmacodynamic and pharmacokinetic properties of these drugs may reduce the incidence of certain adverse reactions and provide greater ease of administration. Each compound must be measured to the needs of each patient, with assessment of the benefit-risk ratio. This ratio must also take into account, the financial impact of a given choice of drug to the potential benefit of that drug in an individual patient.

The clinical observation that β-adrenoceptor blocking drugs are useful for so many different indications demonstrates the importance of the sympathetic nervous system in disease states and the role of the β-adrenoceptors in multiple organ systems. The molecular biology of the β-adrenoceptor itself is being explored. This may shed light on the nature of pharmacologic receptors and their activity.

THE β-ADRENOCEPTOR: CHANGING CONCEPTS

Thirty years ago Ahlquist[63] performed detailed studies in which he thought to characterize the receptors by which catecholamines such as epinephrine and norepinephrine exert their physiologic effects. His studies indicated that there were two major types of receptors: α- and β-adrenoceptors. Adrenergic receptors have since been subclassified into discrete β_1 and β_2[64] as well as α_1 and α_2[65] subtypes. The recent development of radioligand labeling techniques have greatly aided the investigation of adrenoceptors, their molecular properties, and their physiologic regulation.[66]

The older classical concept of adrenoceptors as static entities in cells which simply serve to initiate the chain of events that lead to hormone action is no longer tenable. The newer theory is that the adrenoceptors are subject to a wide variety of controlling influences. The result of these influences is to regulate dynamically the number of adrenoceptors in tissues. These changes in tissue concentration of receptor sites are likely involved in mediating important fluctuations in tissue sensitivity to drug action.[66]

There are significant clinical and therapeutic implications in these new principles. An apparent increase in the number of β-adrenoceptors, and thereby a supersensitivity to agonists, may be induced by chronic exposure to antagonists. This phenomenon was described by Glaubiger and Lefkowitz,[67] and may explain the "propranolol withdrawal effect" which occurs in patients with coronary artery disease upon sudden discontinuation of β-adrenoceptor blocking therapy.[68,69] With prolonged β-adrenoceptor blocker therapy, receptor occupancy by catecholamines would be diminished and the number of available receptors is increased. When the β-adrenoceptor blocker is suddenly withdrawn, an increased pool of receptors would be open to endogenous catecholamines. The resultant adrenergic stimulation may precipitate angina or myocardial infarction.

The effects of thyroid hormone on adrenoceptor numbers in experimental studies may provide at least a partial explanation for the therapeutic efficacy of β-adrenergic blockers in treatment of patients with thyrotoxicosis.[70] The receptor-binding sites have been shown to be increased in hyperthyroidism[70] and decreased in hypothyroidism.[71]

The number of β-adrenoceptors have also been shown to increase with alcohol withdrawal,[72] which may explain the beneficial effects of propranolol for this indication.[73]

The concentrations of β-adrenoceptors in the membrane of mononuclear cells significantly decreases with age.[74] This might explain the progressive resistance to β-adrenoceptor blocker therapy reported with increasing age of the hypertensive population. As shown in a study of Buhler et al.,[75] a good response to β-adrenoceptor blocker therapy occurred in 90 percent of hypertensive patients in their twenties, but the percentage of responders fell progressively with increasing age.

An apparent decrease in β-adrenoceptor sites has been associated with the development of refractoriness or desensitization to endogenous catecholamines, a phenomenon caused by the prolonged exposure of these adrenoceptors to high levels of catecholamines.[76,77] This desensitization phenomenon is not caused by a change in receptor formation or degradation, but rather by catecholamine-induced changes in the conformation of the receptor sites, thus rendering them ineffective. These changes are reversible over a period of hours.

β-Adrenoceptor blocking drugs do not induce desensitization or changes in the conformation of receptors. They do however, block the ability of catecholamines to desensitize.

The new information regarding adrenoreceptors has led to a better understanding of the physiologic and pharmacologic mechanisms that regulate their function. These new concepts concerning adrenoreceptor function and regulation should also increase our understanding of agonist activity in disease states.

THE UNRESOLVED QUESTIONS

In 1958, Powell and Slater[78] discovered dichloroisoprenaline (DCI), the first β-adrenoceptor blocker, and for over 15 years, β-blocking drugs have been utilized in clinical medicine. The efficacy of these agents in a multitude of clinical situations has been well demonstrated. There are, however, many unanswered questions:

1. It is not resolved how β-adrenoceptor receptor blockers reduce elevated blood pressure. The postulated mechanisms include a reduction in cardiac output,[79] an inhibition of renin secretion,[80-85] a reduction in plasma volume,[86] a central neural effect,[87,88] a reduction in peripheral vascular resistance,[89,90] and a resetting of baroreceptor levels.[91,92] The resolution of this question may uncover the etiologic mechanisms of essential hypertension.
2. There is a disparity between the short pharmacokinetic half-life of β-adrenoceptor blockers and the observed length of pharmacologic effects.[93-96] Can β-adrenoceptor blockers be administered to patients in less frequent dosing regimens? Are metabolites important?[97]

3. Can the beneficial effects of β-adrenoceptor blockers in experimental myocardial infarction[98] be extrapolated to patients with acute myocardial infarction? Does chronic β-adrenoceptor blocker therapy provide prophylaxis against myocardial infarctions?[99] Do the antiplatelet actions of some β-adrenoceptor drugs have clinical relevance in myocardial infarction prophylaxis?[100]

4. Do pharmacokinetic differences between β-adrenoceptor blockers[101] have clinical relevance? For example, do drugs with increased lipid solubility and rapid uptake in neural tissue have specific advantages or disadvantages in therapy? Does cardioselectivity or intrinsic sympathomimetic activity provide an advantage in therapy?

5. Do β-adrenoceptor blocking agents with α-adrenergic blocking properties (labetalol)[102, 103] provide any advantage in therapy (i.e., coronary spasm)?

6. The applications of β-adrenoceptor blocking drugs in a wide range of clinical situations suggest that sympathoneuroadrenal inbalances may be an important etiological mechanism in disease. The explanation of why β-adrenergic drugs work in such diverse clinical entities such as anxiety,[30] acne vulgaris,[48] and porphyria[49] may provide insights into the mechanism of disease processes. Perhaps, the ancient Greek physicians were actually talking about sympathoadrenal alterations when they described the "humors in balance"[104] as a prerequisite to health.

CONCLUSION AND SUMMARY

The discovery of the α- and β-adrenoceptor, and the successful attempts to block these receptors, have provided one of the most important scientific advances in clinical medicine. The β-adrenoceptor blocking drugs have been shown to be efficacious for a host of cardiovascular and neuroendocrine indications. The addition of β-blockers with varied pharmacodynamic and pharmacokinetic properties has not influenced therapeutic applications. It has provided pharmacologic alternatives, however, when adverse reactions prohibit the use of a specific drug. It has not been resolved whether the differences in lipid solubility of plasma half-life have any clinical relevance when using these drugs.

The simple concept of competitive pharmacologic inhibition at β-adrenoceptor sites has had revolutionary implications in human therapeutics. Moreover, continued research efforts may further elucidate how sympathoneuroadrenal function can influence disease states. The pioneers in adrenoceptor research have left us with an unfinished puzzle. The task of completing that puzzle, to fit all the pieces together so that the answers to the many unsolved questions can be known, is our legacy.

REFERENCES

1. Prichard BNC, Gillam PMS: The use of propranolol in the treatment of hypertension. Br Med J 2: 725-727, 1964
2. Prichard BNC: Propranolol as an antihypertensive agent. Am Heart J 79: 128-133, 1970
3. Hamer J, Sowton E: Effects of propranolol on exercise tolerance in angina pectoris. Am J Cardiol 18: 354-360, 1966
4. Gillam PMS, Prichard BNC: Propranolol in the therapy of angina pectoris. Am J Cardiol 18: 366-369, 1966
5. Gibson D, Sowton E: The use of beta-adrenergic receptor blocking drugs in dysrhythmias. Progr Cardiovasc Dis 12: 16, 1969
6. Jewitt DE, Mercer CJ, Schillingford JP: Practolol in the treatment of cardiac dysrhythmias due to acute myocardial infarction. Lancet 2: 227, 1969
7. Maroko PR, Braunwald E: Modification of myocardial infarction size after coronary occlusion. Ann Intern Med 79: 720, 1973
8. Frishman WH, Sonnenblick EH: Propranolol therapy in acute myocardial infarction. Cardiovasc Med 2: 311, 1977
9. Cohn JN: Nitroprusside and dissecting aneurysms of aorta. N Engl J Med 295: 567, 1976
10. Wheat MW Jr: Treatment of dissecting aneurysms of the aorta: current status. Prog Cardiovasc Dis 16: 87, 1973
11. Cohen LS, Braunwald E: Amelioration of angina pectoris in idiopathic hypertrophic subaortic stenosis with beta-adrenergic blockade. Circulation 35: 847-851, 1967
12. Sloman G: Propranolol in management of muscular subaortic stenosis. Br Heart J 29: 783-787, 1967
13. Turner JRB: Propranolol in the treatment of digitalis-induced and digitalis-resistant tachycardia. Am J Cardiol 18: 450-457, 1966
14. Winkle RA, Lopes MG, Goodman DS, et al.: Propranolol for patients with mitral valve prolapse. Am Heart J 93: 422, 1977
15. Vincent GM, Abildskov JA, Burgess MJ: Q-T interval syndromes. Progr Cardiovasc Dis 16: 523, 1974
16. Shah PM, Kidd L: Circulatory effects of propranolol in children with Fallot's tetralogy. Observations with isoproterenol infusion, exercise and crying. Am J Cardiol 19: 653-657, 1967
17. Meister SG, Engel TR, Feitosa GS, Helfant RH, Frankl WS: Propranolol in mitral stenosis during sinus rhythm. Am Heart J 94: 685, 1977
18. Bhatia ML, Shrivastava S, Roy SG: Immediate haemodynamic effects of a beta-adrenergic blocking agent — propranolol — in mitral stenosis at fixed heart rates. Br Heart J 34: 638, 1972
19. Stubbs D, Pugh D, Bell H: Combined use of isoproterenol and propranolol in cardiogenic shock. Clin Pharmacol Ther 11: 244-250, 1970
20. Teuscher A, Bossi E, Imhof P, et al.: Effect of propranolol on fetal tachycardia in diabetic pregnancy. Am J Cardiol 42: 304, 1978
21. Furberg C, Morsing C: Adrenergic beta-receptor blockade in neurocirculatory asthenia. Pharmacologia Clinica 1: 168-171, 1969
22. Cumming GR, Mir GH: Effects of propranolol on the resting and exercise hemodynamics of pulmonary stenosis. Can J Physiol Pharmacol 47: 137-142, 1969

23. Guntheroth WG, Kawabor I: Tetrad of Fallot. In Moss AJ, Adams FH, Emmanouilides GC (eds): Heart Disease in Infants, Children, and Adolescents, 2nd ed. Baltimore: Williams and Wilkins. 1977, pp 276–289

24. Bada JL: Treatment of erythromegalia with propranolol. Lancet 2: 412, 1977

25. Oka Y, Frishman W, Becker R, et al.: Clinical pharmacology of the new beta adrenergic blocking drugs. Part 10. Beta-adrenoceptor blockade and coronary artery surgery. Am Heart J 99: 255–270, 1980

26. Fox CA: Reduction in the rise of systolic blood pressure during human coitus by the beta-adrenergic blocking agent propranolol. J Reprod Fertil 22: 587–590, 1970

27. Weber RB, Reinmuth O: The treatment of migraine with propranolol. Neurology 22: 366–369, 1972

28. Strang RR: Clinical trial with a beta-receptor antagonist in Parkinsonism. J Neurol Neurosurg Psychiatr 28: 404–406, 1965

29. Murray TJ: Long-term therapy of essential tremor with propranolol. Can Med Assoc J 115: 892, 1976

30. Granville-Grossman KL, Turner P: The effect of propranolol on anxiety. Lancet 1: 788–790, 1966

31. Brewer C: Beneficial effect of beta-adrenergic blockade on "exam nerves" (letter). Lancet 2: 435, 1972

32. Sellers EM, Degani NC, Silm DH, MacLeod SM: Propranolol-decreased noradrenaline secretion and alcohol withdrawal. Lancet 1: 94–95, 1976

33. Grosz HJ: Narcotic withdrawal symptoms in heroin users treated with propranolol. Lancet 2: 564–566, 1972

34. Rapolt RT, Gay GR, Inaba DS: Propranolol: a specific antagonist to cocaine. Clin Toxicol 10: 265, 1977

35. Linken A: Propranolol for L.S.D.-induced anxiety states (letter). Lancet 2: 1039–1040, 1971

36. Yorkston NJ, Zaki SA, Malik MKU, Morrison RC, Havard CWH: Propranolol in the control of schizophrenic symptoms. Br Med J 4: 633–635, 1974

37. Kirk L, Baastrip PC, Schou M: Propranolol and lithium-induced tremor (letter). Lancet 1: 839, 1972

38. Kales A, Soldatos CR, Cadieux R, et al.: Propranolol in the treatment of narcolepsy. Ann Intern Med 93: 741, 1979

39. Das G, Krieger M: Treatment of thyrotoxic storm with intravenous administration of propranolol. Ann Intern Med 70: 985–988, 1969

40. Lee TC, Coffey RJ, Mackin J, et al.: The use of propranolol in the surgical treatment of thyrotoxic patients. Ann Surg 177: 643–647, 1973

41. Caro JF, Castro JH, Glennon JA: Effect of long-term propranolol administration on parathyroid hormone and calcium concentration in primary hyperparathyroidism. Ann Intern Med 91: 740, 1979

42. Fournier A, Coevoet B, De Fremont JF, et al.: Propranolol therapy for secondary hyperparathyroidism in uraemia. Lancet 2: 50, 1978

43. Blum I, Aderka D, Doron M, Laron Z: Suppression of hypoglycemia by DL- propranolol in malignant insulinoma (letter). N Engl J Med 299: 487, 1978

44. Baker L, Barcai A, Kaye R, et al.: Beta-adrenergic blockade and juvenile diabetes: acute studies and long-term therapeutic trial. J Pediatr 75: 19, 1969

45. Caro JF, Besarab A, Burke JF, Glennon JA: A possible role for propranolol in the treat-

ment of renal osteodystrophy. Lancet 2: 451, 1978

46. Zimmerman T, Kaufman H: Timolol: A beta-adrenergic blocking agent for the treatment of glaucoma. Arch Ophthalmol 95: 601, 1977

47. Prys-Roberts C, Kerr JH, Corbett JL, et al.: Treatment of sympathetic overactivity in tetanus. Lancet 1: 542-545, 1969

48. Cunliff WJ, Cotterill J: The effect of propranolol on acne vulgaris and the rate of sebum excretion. Br J Dermatol 83: 550-551, 1970

49. Douer D, Weinberger A, Pinkhas J, Atsmon A: Treatment of acute intermittent porphyria with large doses of propranolol. JAMA 240: 766, 1978

50. Berk JL, Hagen JF, Beyer WH, et al.: The treatment of endotoxin shock by beta adrenergic blockade. Ann Surg 169: 74-81, 1969

51. Berk JL, Hagen JF, Beyer WH, et al.: The treatment of hemorrhagic shock by beta-adrenergic receptor blockade. Surg Gynecol Obstet 125: 311-318, 1967

52. Kobacz GJ: The role of adrenergic blockade in the treatment of ureteral colic. J Urol 107: 949-951, 1972

53. Khanna OMP: Disorders of micturition. Neuropharmacologic basis and results of drug therapy. Urology 8: 316, 1976

54. Oille WA: Beta adrenergic blockade and the phantom limb (letter). Ann Intern Med 73: 1044-1045, 1970

55. Coyne MJ, Bonorris GG, Chung A, Conley D, Schoenfield LJ: Propranolol inhibits bile acid and fatty acid stimulation of cyclic AMP in human colon. Gastroenterology 73: 971, 1977

56. Lechin F, Van Der Dijs B, Bentolila A, Pena F: The spastic colon syndrome; therapeutic and pathophysiologic considerations. J Clin Pharmacol 17: 431, 1977

57. Mitrani A, Oettinger M, Abinader EG, Sharf M: Use of propranolol in dysfunctional labor. Br J Obstet Gynecol 82: 651, 1975

58. Szerkeres L, Papp J, Forster W: The action of adrenergic beta-receptor blocking agents on susceptibility to cardiac arrhythmias in hypothermia and hypoxia. Experientia 21: 720-722, 1965

59. Moriau M, Noel H, Masure R: Effects of alpha and beta receptor stimulating and blocking agents on experimental disseminated intravascular coagulation. Throm Diath Haemorr 32: 157, 1974

60. Szabuniewicz M, McCrady JD, Camp BJ: Treatment of experimentally induced oleander poisoning. Arch Int Pharmacodyn Ther 189: 12-21, 1971

61. Thadani U, Davidson C, Singleton W, Taylor S: Comparison of the immediate effects of five beta-adrenoceptor blocking drugs in angina pectoris. N Engl J Med 300: 750, 1979

62. Frishman W, Silverman R: Clinical Pharmacology of the new beta adrenergic blocking drugs. Part 3. Comparative clinical experience and new therapeutic applications. Am Heart J 98: 119, 1979

63. Ahlquist RP: A study of the adrenotropic receptors. Am J Physiol 153: 586, 1948

64. Lands AM, Arnold A, McAuliff JP, Ludena FP, Brown TG Jr.: Differentiation of receptor systems activated by sympathomimetic amines. Nature 214: 597, 1967

65. Berthelsen S, Pettinger WA: A functional basis for classification of α-adrenergic receptors. Life Sci 21: 595, 1977

66. Lefkowitz RJ: Direct binding sights of adrenergic receptors: biochemical, physiologic, and clinical implications. Ann Intern Med 91: 450, 1979

67. Glaubiger G, Lefkowitz RJ: Elevated beta-adrenergic receptor number after chronic

propranolol treatment. Biochem Biophys Res Commun 78: 720, 1977
68. Shand DG, Wood AJJ: Propranolol withdrawal syndrome — why? Circulation 58: 202, 1978
69. Alderman EL, Coltart DJ, Wettach GE, Harrison DC: Coronary artery syndromes after sudden propranolol withdrawal. Ann Intern Med 81: 625, 1974
70. Williams LT, Lefkowitz RJ, Watanabe AM, Hathaway DR, Besch HR Jr: Thyroid hormone regulation of β-adrenergic receptor number. J Biol Chem 252: 2787, 1977
71. Banerjee SP, Kung LS: β-adrenergic receptors in the rat heart: effects of thyroidectomy. Eur J Pharmacol 43: 207, 1977
72. Banerjee SP, Sharma VK, Khanna JM: Alteration in β-adrenergic receptor binding during ethanol withdrawal. Nature 276: 407, 1978
73. Sellers EM, Degani NC, Silm DH, MacLeod SM: Propranolol-decreased noradrenaline secretion and alcohol withdrawal. Lancet 1: 94, 1976
74. Schoken DD, Roth GS: Reduced β-adrenergic receptor concentrations in aging man. Nature 267: 856, 1977
75. Bühler FR, Bukart F, Benno LE, et al.: Antihypertensive beta-blocking action as related to renin and age. A pharmacological tool to identify pathogenic mechanisms in essential hypertension. Am J Cardiol 36: 653, 1975
76. Lefkowitz RJ: β-adrenergic receptors: recognition and regulation. N Engl J Med 295: 323, 1976
77. Mukherjee C, Lefkowitz RJ: Regulation of beta-adrenergic receptors in isolated frog erythrocyte membranes. Mol Pharmacol 13: 291, 1977
78. Powell CE, Slater IH: Blocking of inhibitory adrenergic receptors by a trichloro-analogue of isoproterenol. J Pharmacol Exp Ther 122: 480, 1958
79. Frolich ED, Tarazi RC, Dustan HP, Page IH: The paradox of β-adrenergic blockade in hypertension. Circulation 37: 417, 1968
80. Michelkis AM, McAllister RG: The effect of chronic adrenergic receptor blockade on plasma renin activity in man. J Clin Endocrinol Metab 34: 386, 1972
81. Winer N, Chokshi DS, Yoom MS, Freedman AD: Adrenergic receptor mediation of renin secretion. J Clin Endocrinol Metab 29: 1168, 1969
82. Buhler FR, Laragh JH, Baer JL, Vaughan ED Jr, Brunner HR: Propranolol inhibition of renin secretion, a specific approach to diagnosis and treatment of renin dependent hypertensive diseases. N Engl J Med 287: 1209, 1972
83. Castenfors J, Johnsson H, Oro L: Effect of alprenolol on blood pressure and plasma renin activity in hypertensive patients. Acta Med Scand 193: 189, 1973
84. Zech PY, Labeeuw M, Pozet N, et al.: Response to atenolol in arterial hypertension in relation to renal function, pharmacokinetics and renin activity. Postgrad Med J 53 (Suppl 3): 134, 1977
85. von Bahr C, Collste P, Frisk-Holmberg M, et al.: Plasma levels and effects of metoprolol on blood pressure, adrenergic receptor blockade and plasma renin activity in essential hypertension. Clin Pharmacol Ther 20: 130, 1976
86. Tarazi RC, Frolich ED, Dustan HP: Plasma volume changes with long-term beta-adrenergic blockade. Am Heart J 82: 720, 1971
87. Dollery CT, Lewis PJ: Central hypotensive effect of propranolol. Postgrad Med J 52 (Suppl 4): 116, 1976
88. Srivatsava RL, Kulshrestha VK, Singh N, Bhargava K: Central cardiovascular effect of extracerebroventricular propranolol. Eur J Pharmacol 21: 222, 1973

208 FRISHMAN

89. Atterhög JH, Duner H, Pernow B: Hemodynamic effect of long-term treatment with pindolol in essential hypertension with special reference to resistance and capacitance vessels of the forearm. Acta Med Scand 202: 517, 1977
90. Birkenhäger WH, DeLeeuw PW, Wester A, et al.: Therapeutic effects of β-adrenoceptor blocking agents in hypertension. In Frisk P, et al. (eds): Advances in Internal Medicine and Pediatrics, Vol. 39. Berlin: Springer-Verlag, 1977, p. 117
91. Prichard BNC, Gillam PMS: Treatment of hypertension with propranolol. Br Med J 1: 7, 1969
92. Dunlop D, Shanks RG: Inhibition of the carotid sinus reflex by chronic administration of propranolol. Br J Pharmacol 36: 132, 1967
93. Berglund G, Andersson O, Hansson L, Orlander R: Propranolol given twice daily in hypertension. Acta Med Scand 194: 513, 1973
94. Hansson L, Orlander R, Åberg H: Twice daily propranolol treatment of hypertension. Lancet 2: 713, 1971
95. Wilson M, Morgan G, Morgan T: The effect on blood pressure of β-adrenoreceptor blocking drugs given once daily. Clin Sci Mol Med 51: 527s, 1976
96. Vedin A, Wilhelmsson C, Werkö L: Comparative study of alprenolol and methyldopa in previously untreated hypertension. Br Heart J 35: 1285, 1973
97. Frishman W: Clinical Pharmacology of the new beta adrenergic blocking drugs. Part 1. Pharmacodynamic and pharmacokinetic properties. Am Heart J 97: 663, 1979
98. Maroko PR, Braunwald E: Modification of myocardial infarction size after coronary occlusion. Ann Intern Med 79: 720, 1973
99. Multicentre International Study: Improvement in prognosis of myocardial infarction by long-term beta-adrenoceptor blockade using practolol. Br Med J 1: 837, 1976
100. Frishman WH, Weksler B, Christodoulou J, Smithen C, Killip T: Reversal of abnormal platelet aggregability and change in exercise tolerance in patients with angina pectoris following oral propranolol. Circulation 50: 887, 1974
101. Johnsson G, Regardh CG: Clinical pharmacokinetics of β-adrenoreceptor blocking drugs. Clin Pharmacokin 1: 233, 1976
102. Farmer JB, Kennedy I, Levy GP, Marshall RJ: Pharmacology of AH 5158: a drug which blocks both alpha and β-adrenoceptors. Br Symbol
103. Frishman W, Halprin S: Clinical pharmacology of the new beta adrenergic blocking drugs. Part 7. New horizons in beta-adrenoceptor blockade therapy: labetalol. Am Heart J 97: 663, 1979
104. Lyons AS, Petrucelli RJ: Medicine. New York, Abrams, 1976, p 251

APPENDIX

Drug Interactions That May Occur with β-Adrenoceptor Blocking Drugs*

Drug	Possible Effects	Precautions
Aminophylline	Mutual inhibition	Observe patient's response
Antidiabetic agents	Enhanced hypoglycemia: hypertension	Monitor for altered diabetic response
Calcium channel inhibitors (e.g., Verapimil)	Potentiation of bradycardia, myocardial depression, and hypotension	Avoid use, although few patients show ill effects
Clonidine	Hypertension during clonidine withdrawal	Monitor for hypertensive response; withdraw β-blocker before withdrawing clonidine
Digitalis glycosides	Potentiation of bradycardia	Observe patient's response; interactions may benefit angina patients with abnormal ventricular function
Epinephrine	Hypertension; bradycardia	Administer epinephrine cautiously; cardioselective β-blocker may be safer
Ergot alkaloids	Excessive vasoconstriction	Observe patient's response; few patients show ill effects
Glucagon	Inhibition of hyperglycemic effect	Monitor for reduced response
Halofenate	Reduced β-blocking activity; production of propranolol withdrawal rebound syndrome	Observe for impaired response to β-blockade
Indomethacin	Inhibition of antihypertensive response to β-blockade	Observe patient's response
Isoproterenol	Mutual inhibition	Avoid concurrent use or choose cardiac selective β-blocker
Levodopa	Antagonism of levodopa's hypotensive and positive inotropic effects	Monitor for altered response; interaction may have favorable results
Methyldopa	Hypertension during stress	Monitor for hypertensive episodes

(continued)

Drug Interactions That May Occur with β-Adrenoceptor Blocking Drugs* (cont.)

Drug	Possible Effects	Precautions
Monoamine oxidase inhibitors	Uncertain, theoretical	Manufacturer of propranolol considers concurrent use contraindicated
Phenothiazines	Additive hypotensive effects	Monitor for altered response especially with high doses of phenothiazine
Phenylpropanolamine	Severe hypertensive reaction	Avoid use, especially in hypertension controlled by both methyldopa and β-blockers
Phenytoin	Additive cardiac depressant effects	Administer IV phenytoin with great caution
Quinidine	Additive cardiac depressant effects	Observe patient's response; few patients show ill effects
Reserpine	Excessive sympathetic blockade	Observe patient's response
Tubocurarine	Enhanced neuromuscular blockade	Observe response in surgical patients, especially after high doses of propranolol

*Adapted from Hansten PD: Drug Interactions, 4th ed. Philadelphia, Lea & Febiger, 1979, p 13

INDEX

β-Adrenoceptor blocking drugs (*cont.*)
  antihypertensive action, 35–39
    variation in, 38–39
  anxiety, therapy for, 49–50
  bronchoconstriction induced by, 26
  carcinogenicity of, 66–67
  cardioprotective effect in management
    of myocardial infarction, 128
  cardioselective, 6–7, 22
    advantages of, 6–7
    partial agonist activity of, 18
    therapeutic implications of, 20
  cardiovascular indications for, 199
  cautions for use of, 27
  central nervous system and, 15–16, 64
  changing concepts of, 201–202
  chemical structures of, 3–5
  chest pains and, 42
  clearance, 10–11
  clinical indications, common, 35
  clinical observation of, 200–201
  clinical situations, influence of, 67–68
  clinical trials of, 59–61
  contraindications of systemic use of, 51
  definition of, 4
  development of, 2
  differences in pharmacologic
    properties among, 3
  differing from propranolol, 141
  drug interactions with, 209–210
  elimination characteristics of orally
    administered, 10
  FDA approved, 2, 200
  half-life of, 89
  hemodynamic effects, long-term, 48
  how to choose, 67–68
  hypertrophic cardiomyopathy, therapy
    for, 48
  long acting, 163–70
  mechanisms of prophylactic action of,
    128
  migraine prophylaxis, use for, 49
  myocardial infarction, therapy for, 49
  narcotic and alcohol withdrawal,
    clinical effects in, 50–51
  negative inotropism of, 123
  newer applications of, 47–49

β-Adrenoceptor blocking drugs (*cont.*)
  noncardiovascular indications for, 200
  perspective, 199–208
  pharmacodynamic properties
    and cardiac effects of, 22
    and noncardiac effects of, 25
    and pharmacokinetic properties, 1–14
  pharmacokinetic parameters, 9
  pharmacologic properties, summary
    of, 80
  potency of, 2–3
  prophylactic effect in management of
    myocardial infarction, 128
  prophylactic use in angina pectoris, 39
  questions, unresolved, 202–203
  rebound effect of, 63
  schizophrenia, therapy for, 50
  self-poisoning with, 73–95
  stereoisomers of, 4
  structural formulas of, 5
  therapeutic and toxic dose levels and, 89
  therapeutic indications, 15, 49–51
  tremor, therapy for, 49
  tumorigenicity of, 2
  withdrawal of, 62–63
Adrenoceptors
  distribution of, 1
  α-receptors, 1
  β-receptors
    β_1-receptors, 1
    β_2-receptors, 1
    bronchial and vascular, 6
    cardiac, 6, 19
    change in concentrations with age, 202
    classical concepts of, 201
    effect of alcohol withdrawal, 201
    effects of thyroid hormone on, 201
    in myocardial cells, effects of
      stimulation of, 18
  types of, 1
Agonists, supersensitivity to, 201
Ahlquist, R.P., 1, 171, 201
Airway resistance, 26
Albert Einstein College of Medicine
    Committee on Use of Human
    Subjects in Research, approval of,
    136